DISTRICT OF VERMONT, TO WIT:

BE IT REMEMBERED, That on the fifth day of November, in the forty-eighth year of the Independence of the United States of America, JONATHAN MORRISON, of the said district, hath deposited in this office, the title of a Book, the right whereof he claims as proprietor, in the words following, to wit:

L. S.

"THE AMERICAN BOTANIST, AND FAMILY PHYSICIAN. By JOHN MONROE. Two Volumes in one."

In conformity to the Act of the Congress of the United States, entitled, "An act for the encouragement of learning, by securing the copies of Maps, Charts, and Books, to the Authors and Proprietors of such copies, during the times therein mentioned.

JESSE GOVE,
Clerk of the District of Vermont.

A true copy of record,
Examined and sealed by me,
J. GOVE, *Clerk.*

PREFACE.

TO THE PUBLIC.

The author of the following sheets is a native of New-Hampshire, but now resides in the northerly part of Vermont; where he has been for a number of years engaged in the practice of physic;—and as health is the foundation of all the enjoyments of life, the preservation of it (next to our eternal well-being in the world towards which we are making rapid advances) demands our most serious attention;—for if possessed of all that this perishing world could afford, without this inestimable blessing, our conditions would be miserable.

It is clear as the sun at noon day, that nature has provided in her minerals, animals, and vegetables, an effectual remedy, if administered in season, for all the disorders incident to the human system. Of the two latter, the author has treated more particularly in the following work, omitting the minerals; which, on account of their poisonous quality, ought, in his humble opinion, to be laid aside.

Under these considerations, he here offers to the public a work, in which, after treating in a botanical way of the animal and vegetable productions of the climate, he has taken up each disorder separately, and endeavored to point out to his fellow creatures the means by which they may be successfully met at every point, and with due perseverance, and the blessing of Heaven, effectually overcome.

For the attainment of this object, he has travelled; to this end he has labored; and for years has he plied himself in the wilds of America, among the natives of the forest, where he has undergone all the horrors and deprivations incident to savage life, in order to collect, and bring together that knowledge which should be instrumental in saving the lives and preserving the health of his fellow creatures.

PREFACE.

Whilst among the Indians, the Author was a particular intimate and confidant of a native Indian, who had been instructed in all the arts of civilized life, and had received the advantages of a liberal and polite education, being regularly bred a physician in the medical department of the Pennsylvania University, established at Philadelphia; at once the most flourishing and respectable institution of the kind in the United States, and hardly excelled by any in Europe. Whilst with this Indian, the Author had not only an opportunity of learning the Indian methods of treating disorders, and the medical virtues of the vegetable kingdom, but likewise of gaining much literary and scientific knowledge.

Previous to this, however, he had studied the medical art with several physicians, according to the methods then in vogue, and spent much time in reading different authors, among which were Culpepper, Bœrhaave, &c.—and after returning from the Indians, the Author spent two years and a half in study with a German physician of great repute in order to perfect himself in the knowledge of chemical operations, and the anatomy of the human frame.

And after devoting above seven years to travel and study, during which period he travelled through nine of the United States for the purpose of collecting an account of the most recent discoveries among the Indians, English, and Germans, and studied with the most noted and eminent physicians of the day, he is mistaken if he has not compressed within the compass of this work a greater number of valuable discoveries in the medical art than has ever been brought to light at any former period of time since the world began.

THE AMERICAN BOTANIST,

AND

FAMILY PHYSICIAN.

VOL. I.

ADDER'S TONGUE.

THE bruised leaves of this plant are good in fresh wounds and internal bruises. Cataplasms of the same are of great service in the hæmorrhoides.

AGRIMONY—SWEET.

This herb is of a cooling and astringent quality. Infusions of the plant are of great service in fevers, dysenteries, and disorders of the stomach.

ALDER—SPECKLED.

It is stomachic and anthelmintic. It makes a good bitter, and has been used in consumptions, coughs, and extreme debility.

ANGELICA.

This herb is carminitive and discutient. Infusions of it expel wind—help flatulent cholics; and the fresh roots, applied externally, discuss inflammatory tumors, and excite spitting.

APPLE TREE—SWEET.

The buds of the sweet Apple Tree, infused in rum or cider, are excellent for correcting the humors, and sweetening the blood and juices, especially in the spring of the year.

ARSMART—BITING.

This excellent herb, of which too much cannot

be said, is diobstruent, stimulant, diuretic and emmenegogic.

It removes obstructions, helps the gravel; and in recent colds, is not exceeded by any other herb yet discovered. It is likewise a great preventive of fevers, if administered in season.

ARTICHOKE.

This plant is a powerful diuretic.

The juice, mixed with an equal quantity of white wine, powerfully promotes urine. The roots make a more wholesome pickle than cucumbers.

ASH—WHITE.

The bark is called astringent and sudorific. Both the inner bark, and its watery extract, have been given in intermitting fevers and consumptions. with success. In decoction, it sweetens the blood and juices; and the internal and external use of the juice that issues out of the wood, while burning, has been celebrated as a cure for a cancer.

ASH—PRICKLY.

The bark of this tree is a great purifier of the blood and juices.

An ounce pulverized and digested in a pint of brandy is an excellent medicine in rheumatisms, and for the intermitting fever and ague.

Captain Carver says, that the Indians esteemed a decoction of the bark of the root a good remedy in a violent gonorrhea; and that it has sometimes cured one in a few days.

ASAFŒTIDA.

Asafœtida is the strongest of the fœtid gums, and of frequent use in hysteric, and different kinds of nervous complaints. It is likewise of considerable efficacy in flatulent cholies; and for promoting all the fluid secretions of either sex. Many virtues, however, have been attributed to this medicine, which, at present, are not expected from it.*

BALM.

This has been extolled by many authors; yet I have never found it of any great use. It is, however, a weak corroborant.

BALSAM OF FIR.

This balsam has been much celebrated for the cure of wounds and bruises: but I have almost invariably found it to be of too irritating a quality. It generally proves diuretic.

BALSAM RACASARI.

This is one of the most powerful balsams; possessing all the virtues attributed to balsam Ca-

* Vide Edinburgh Dispensatory.

pivi, and in a much higher degree. It is excellent in plaisters, and cures wounds, without leaving any eschar. Taken internally, it removes rheumatic and sciatic complaints ;—and, in fact, no family ought to do without this most valuable remedy.

BARBERRY.

The bark of the roots is somewhat astringent. The inner bark of the tree is gently purgative. An ounce of the inner bark, infused in a pint of boiling water, is esteemed a good remedy in the jaundice. Strong decoctions may likewise be used with success in the same disorder.

BARLEY.

The hulled grain makes a wholesome diet in fevers, and many other disorders ; being more cooling and less cloying than any other grain.

BAY BERRY BUSH.

The leaves and berries of this bush are stomachic and emmenagogic, anti-hysteric, and slightly diuretic. They are good in hysterical complaints, menstrual obstructions, and to correct gross humors.

BEAR.

The flesh of this animal is eaten by the Indians, without any farinaceous root or plant to absorb the grosser parts. The oil is less cloying than that of any other animal. It is used to advantage by the Indian women for a considerable time before delivery. It is likewise of great service in phthisics, quinsy, stiff joints, &c. The gall is also good in stiff joints, sprains, and rheumatisms.

BEECH TREE.

The bark of this tree is a great styptic and astringent.

The juice which collects upon the inside of the bark of this tree, in the month of June, mixed with an equal quantity of fresh butter or lard, makes an excellent salve for a burn.

BEET—COMMON.

Their juice is purifying to the blood and juices; but after the juice is boiled out, they are hard to digest, and afford but little nourishment.

BISTORTA.*

It is a great styptic and tonic. It is also a carminative.

Decoctions of the root open obstructions; and outwardly, in fomentations, they help stubborn ulcers of the legs, and cure cutaneous disorders.

BITTER SWEET.

This plant is a resolvent, discutient, diuretic, emmenagogue, and anti-venereal.

* Called also Birthwort, Benjamin, &c.

It opens obstructions, resolves and discusses hard tumors; and is good in jaundice, scurvy, obstructions of the menses, and lues-Venerea.

BLACK BERRY.

The fruit is cooling, and eaten raw, or in milk, makes a very wholesome diet.

The roots of the bush are astringent, and good in dysenteries and diarrhœa.

BLACK CHERRY.

The bark of this tree is an emmenagogue, and anodyne. Infused in rum, it makes an excellent bitter in jaundice.

BLESSED THISTLE.

Light infusions of the plant have been esteemed good in loss of appetite and indigestion.

It removes obstructions, and raises insensible perspiration; but in large doses it proves emetic.

BLOOD ROOT.

This root is a powerful stimulant, and a violent emetic and cathartic; but given in small doses, and carefully used, it is an excellent remedy for the canker, and cleansing ulcers in the internal viscera.

An external application of the powdered roots, destroys fungus flesh, and heals sores of long standing.

BROOK LIME.

This is a low plant, common in little rivulets and ditches of standing water. The leaves remain all winter; but are in greatest perfection in the spring.

Its juice taken freely is useful in hot constitutions and the hemorrhoids.

BRAKE—HOG, OR FEMALE FERN.

This plant is discutient, diuretic and sudorific. It discusses hard tumors, removes obstructions; and, in strong decoction, it is an excellent medicine in dysenteries, consumptions and rickets.

BRAKE—BLACK TOPPED.

The Author was informed, while among the Indians, that they once cured a captive of the rheumatism, when he had been helpless a number of days, by sweating him with these brakes, in the following manner:

They placed a great quantity of these brakes upon a flat stone, after it had been heated; and after placing him upon the brakes, they covered him with a blanket, giving him decoctions of the root in the mean time.

BURDOCK.

This is a great carminative; and although despised by many as a cumbersome plant, it is one of the finest productions of which our country can boast. Decoctions of the root open obstructions—sweeten the animal fluids, and promote sweat and urine. It is, likewise, good in rheumatic and venereal disorders, dry coughs, asthma and pleurisy; acting without irritation. An infusion of the pulverized seeds in rum, helps disorders of the breast and lungs. The leaves, applied to the soles of the feet, make a revulsion from the head.

BUTTER NUT.

The bark of this tree, rightly prepared, constitutes one of the best and safest physics ever known. It is a great cleanser of the lungs; good in phthisics, and all other disorders of the like nature. The oil of the nuts is an excellent application for sore nipples of women, and almost all other humors.

BORAGE.

This is a cooling and wholesome herb, and makes a good drink in fevers and inflammatory complaints. It is cultivated in gardens, mostly for culinary purposes.

BUTTER MILK.

That made by churning new milk makes a cooling and wholesome diet, and is good in consumptions, weakness, loss of appetite; and, drank freely, proves diuretic.

CABBAGE.

This plant is attenuant, laxative, and anti-scorbutic.

Decoctions of the red cabbage soften acrid humors—promote expectoration; and are good in hoarseness and disorders of the breast. The leaves, applied externally, promote the discharge of blisters.

CHAMOMILE.

This valuable herb, of which too much cannot be said, is a powerful antiseptic, antispasmodic, and anodyne.

It increases the force of the circulation, and invigorates the system in general—softens and discusses hard tumors—resists putrefaction, and eases pain. It is good in consumptions, recent colds, and putrid disorders. In external applications, it is good for weak eyes and other humors.

CANKER ROOT.

This is good in sore mouth, and canker: but if it has any other medical virtue, it is unknown to the Author.

CARAWAY.

The seeds are stomachic and carminative. They expel wind—strengthen the stomach—ease pain; and are good in flatulent cholic.

CARROT—WILD.

This root is powerfully stimulant, and a great emmenagogue.

It helps recent colds—removes obstructions—promotes the menses, and secretions in general.

CASTOR—BEAVER.

This is an antispasmodic, emmenagogue, and antihysteric.

It is good in menstrual obstructions, hysterical complaints, and a celebrated medicine in the palsy, epilepsy, convulsions, &c. But the Author has found but little benefit from the use of it in the last mentioned disorders.

CASTOR OIL BUSH.

From the seeds of the bush, (which resembles in colour and shape the stick, called Ricinus) is expressed the oil called castor oil, which, although very celebrated physic, the author has found to be greatly inferior to many others, and not altogether to be depended upon.

CEDAR—RED.

The oil, obtained by distilling the shavings of this cedar, is a very valuable medicine in rheumatism and stiff joints.

CEDAR—WHITE.

To this belongs all the virtues of Cedar Red, with this addition: the oil obtained by distillation is an extraordinary medicine in rheumatism and hemorrhoids.

CELENDYNE.

This is emollient, discutient, anodyne and antiscorbutic.

It is good in jaundice and hemorrhoids. The clear juice extirpates warts, and cures ringworms.

CELERY—*vulgarly called* LOVAGE.

This plant has been esteemed a great emmenagogue by some: but its virtues, in this respect, are not much to be depended on.

COLD WATER ROOT.

This plant is diuretic;—good in gravel, strangury, and other uterine complaints.

Infusions of the herb and root purify the blood and juices, and prevent fevers, if administered in season.

COHUSH—WHITE.

Although no writer has described the virtues of this plant, the Author has found it serviceable in many disorders.

It strengthens the system in general, and is good in fluor albus, menstrual obstructions, and other female disorders. Taken in decoction, it prevents taking cold, when exposed: and, indeed, every lady, of whatever grade, should not hesitate to drop a courtesy as she passes by this genteel herb.

CUMFREY.

Of the consolidating virtues of this plant, many ridiculous stories have been related by authors. It is serviceable in diarrhœas and dysenteries; but it is not much used in the present practice.

CONVULSION ROOT.

This root is anti-spasmodic, and nervine. It is good in convulsions, cramps, and hypochondria.

CORIANDER.

The seeds of this plant are a great carminative; and help flatulent cholics.

COW PARSNIP.

The roots are carminative and anti-hysteric. They remove hysterical complaints, flatulence, vertigo, dimness of sight, trembling, and anxiety—help the appetite, and have cured the epilepsy.

COWSLIP.

The flowers of this herb are anti-spasmodic and anodyne.

They help nervous complaints, allay cramps and spasms—ease pain, and strengthen the system in general.

They are good in menstrual obstructions, apoplexy, vertigo and palsy.

COOL WORT.

This herb is good in consumptions; and makes a very cooling and salutary drink in fevers. It is good in tickling coughs, hoarseness, internal heats, and inflammatory disorders.

CRANBERRY.

These berries make a very wholesome and agreeable tart, which is good in fevers, and helps the appetite.

CUCUMBER.

This fruit is cultivated in gardens for culinary uses. It is hard to digest, and affords but little nourishment. It is of so cold a nature that it ought to be seasoned with salt, vinegar, and pepper, when eaten. It is, however, good in hot bilious habits.

CROW'S FOOT.

The roots and leaves of this plant have an acrid and fiery taste: and, according to Dr. Stearns, they prove deleterious, when taken internally, even when so far freed from their causticity, by boiling, as to discover no ill quality to the palate.

The leaves, applied externally, blister the part, and have been used for this purpose.

CULVER'S ROOT.

It grows three or four feet high;—has a green root, of a darkish hue on the outside, and brown within, somewhat in the form of the root of scabious. The flowers are whitish, and resemble, in form, the top of a corn stalk.

It is good in scrofulous complaints;—operates as a cathartic; and may be taken in decoction, or in substance.

CUDWEED.

The clear juice of this herb is said to cure warts, remove freckles, sun-burns, &c.

CURRANT.

The fruit is refrigerant and antalkaline;—good

in fevers, and all cases where vegetable acids are necessary.

Infusions of the prunes have likewise been used in fevers, with success.

An agreeable wine is obtained by adding to the juice of red currants, an equal quantity of water, and a pound of sugar to every quart of currant juice. After this has stood a year, it is fit for use.

CIDER.

Good cider is cordial and anti-scorbutic, and a wholesome liquor for most constitutions. It is good in scorbutic and melancholy habits; and in many cases preferable to wine.

DANDELION.

This plant is diuretic and sudorific. It helps the jaundice; and is good in consumptions, weakness, loss of appetite and debility. It is a great corrector of humors; but it should be used for a long time.

DRAGON ROOT.

This root is a powerful stimulant, diuretic, and diaphoretic.

It attenuates the viscid fluids—stimulates the solids, and promotes the natural secretions in general.

It is good in cold, languid, phlegmatic habits; in relaxations, and weakness of the stomach; loss of appetite; intermitting diseases; hysteric and hypochondriac affections; catarrhs; cachexy; rheumatic pains; and obstinate head-aches.

DOCK—YELLOW.

This is astringent and agglutinant.

The juice is a fine application for cancers; and the roots are celebrated as a cure for the itch.

DOCK—CONSUMPTION.

This is of a balsamic quality.

It purifies the blood and juices; and is good in

phthisics, consumptions and coughs; but it ought to be continued for a long time. Dr. Stearns informs that a poultice of the root cures the king's-evil.

DEVIL'S BIT.

This plant has been used with success in gargles; for inflammations of the fauces, and venereal ulcers of the mouth and throat; and the juice, internally, for malignant ulcers, bubos, carbuncles, and epileptic fits.

DOG.

This creature is the most faithful and grateful of domestic animals. The oil is good in burns and scalds.

DOG MACKIMUS.

The bark, berries, and leaves of the shrub are

good in jaundice, consumptions, fluor albus, and strangurine complaints.

It removes obstructions of the internal viscera. The dried bark is smoked for the tooth and head-ache, and chewed for the tooth-ache by the Indians.

EARTH WORMS.

These worms are dug out of wet, sandy land; and by some are called *angle* worms. They are excellent in heart burn, epilepsy, cramp convulsions; and a sovereign remedy for stiff joints. One half pint, dissolved in one pound of sugar, is an Indian medicine in consumptions, coughs, internal weakness, and dropsical complaints.

EGGS

Are highly nutritious, and one of the greatest strengtheners known. An egg, taken in spirit every morning in cases of extreme debility, has often performed an effectual cure.

ELECAMPANE.

The roots, according to Dr. Stearns, are expectorant, attenuant, laxative, stomachic, diuretic, diaphoretic, and alexipharmic. But I have found it of very little use.

ELM—SWEET.

The inner bark of the tree is emollient; and a drink of the same, used freely, is good in internal weakness and fluor albus. It has likewise been used in affections of the lungs, burns and scalds. But its virtues, I think, are not to be depended on.

FEATHER FEW.

This herb is stomachic, emmenegogic, and anti-venereal. When properly prepared, it makes an excellent bitter.

FENNEL.

The roots of this plant are aperient and diuretic;—the seeds carminative. Decoctions of the root help the stone in the kidney and bladder, and promote urine. The seeds expel wind, and help nausea, and loathing of food.

FENNEL—SWEET.

According to Dr. Stearns, the seeds are carminative and stomachic.

They attenuate viscid humors; expel wind; help the stomach; and promote sweat and urine.

FERN—MEADOW.

This vegetable has been neglected by almost all writers. But I have found it to possess all the virtues of the other ferns; and in a much higher degree.

It is a powerful anthelmintic, and a great carminative.

It is good in weakness of stomach; loss of appetite and indigestion.

It is a great corrector of internal humors; and often a powerful remedy in cases of extreme debility.

FERN—SWEET.

The bark of the root is a weak anthelmintic: but it is not possessed of so great virtues as has generally been supposed. It makes, however, a good beer.

FEVER BUSH.

This vegetable is used by the Indians with success in all cases of inflammation.

It is good in low fevers, weakness of stomach, and loss of appetite.

FIVE FINGERS.

This is a trailing plant, which grows wild in pastures in many parts of America.

The roots are good in colliquative diarrhœas; intermitting and acute fevers; and gargarisms for strengthening the gums.

FLAG—CATTAIL.

This is good in internal heats; dysentery, and strangury. It likewise makes a cooling and salutary drink in fevers. Cataplasms of the root are excellent in burns.

FLAG—SWEET.

This is an agreeable stomachic, aromatic and carminative.

It strengthens the stomach; expels wind; resolves obstructions, and promotes the secretions in general.

It purifies the blood, and has been used to keep off epidemic diseases.

FLAG—BLUE.

This is a powerful emmenagogue, and anti-venereal. The roots are likewise diuretic: but, if taken in large doses, it irritates the throat.

FLAG—YELLOW.

The roots are a strong cathartic; and often produce copious evacuations, after jalep gamboge, and other strong cathartics, prove ineffectual.

FLAX—COMMON.

The seeds are a powerful emmenagogue. The expressed oil is an excellent remedy in burns and scalds.

The seeds have been celebrated in defluxions of the lungs; and all disorders of the like nature:

but the Author has generally found it to be a deceitful medicine, and not at all to be depended on.

FOX GLOVE.

This plant grows wild in gravelly grounds. It has been celebrated by many in disorders of the lungs, and many others. But I have found it in all cases to prove hurtful to the human system, and destructive to the lungs; and of a very poisonous and irritating quality.

GARGET, or STOKE.

This plant is powerfully stimulant, emetic, and cathartic.

The roots, applied to the feet, make a revulsion from the head.

The juice of the berries, put into a pewter dish, and dried away in the sun to the consistence of salve, is beneficial in cancers, and cancer humors.

An infusion of the berries in brandy is an Indian medicine for the rheumatism. An external application of the sliced roots, promotes the discharge of foul ulcers; and a powder of the same is good in venereal taints.

GARLIC—GARDEN.

This is stimulant, diuretic, and anthelmintic.

The juice, mixed with brandy, and applied to the head, is good in obstinate head-aches; but not equal to wild leeks.

It is good in dropsies; and, applied to the soles of the feet, it makes a revulsion from the head.

GINSENG.

This is a great stomachic.

Decoctions of the root are good in cold, phlegmatic habits; but hurtful in hot, bilious constitutions; it being a hot and pungent root.

In China, it is resorted to as a last remedy in all disorders.

It is destructive in the piles, and has proved immediately fatal.

GENTIAN—AMERICAN.

The root is of a pale yellowish color—jointed and marked with various knots and circles, like Ipecacuanha.

It makes a good bitter; and may serve as a substitute for the Peruvian bark.

GOLD THREAD.

This is excellent in canker, and sore mouth; and is used with success in gargles. It makes an excellent bitter.

GOLDEN ROD.

This herb grows wild in waste pasture grounds, and by the side of fields.

Decoctions of the herb are excellent in weakness and debility. It is a great cleanser of the internal viscera; and a preventive of consumptions and dropsies.

Of it there are two kinds: the largest of these is the strongest.

GOOSE.

The flesh of this fowl makes a very wholesome diet.

The oil is a good remedy in phthisics; and an effectual cure for corns: but the feathers are very hurtful to those who lie upon them, in the phthisic.

GOOSE GRASS, or CLIVERS.

It is a slender, rough vine, growing in moist land, by the sides of brooks and rivers, and sticking to whatever it touches.

It is a great diuretic; and has been used in dropsies; but it is hurtful to the urinary organs.

GOOSEBERRY BUSH.

The unripe fruit is acrid and astringent, and makes a very wholesome and agreeable tart.

A decoction of the prunes is a very cooling and salutary drink in fevers.

GOURD.

This is cultivated in gardens.

The seeds, infused in brandy, are good in strangurine complaints.

GRAPE VINE.

This is a powerful diuretic.

The juice obtained from this vine in the spring of the year, by tapping, stops the operation of spirituous liquor.

GRASS—KNOT.

This is a cooling, diuretic, and astringent plant.

It is good in dysenteries, fluxes, and uterine complaints.

GROUND IVY.

The juice is good in weakness, jaundice, the beginning of consumptions ; and a great purifier of the blood and juices.

In decoction, it removes obstructions ; and is good in ulcerations of the lungs, kidneys, and laxity and debility of the internal viscera.

GROUND NUT.

It grows in many parts of New-England, and is about the size of a nutmeg.

It is good in strangury, diabetes, and bloody urine.

GROUND PINE.

According to Dr. Stearns, the leaves are aperient ; corroborant ; nervine ; attenuant ; diuretic, and emmenagogic : and good in gout ; rheumatism ; palsy ; suppression of urine, and uterine obstructions.

GUINEA PEPPER;—

Called also RED PEPPER. It is a powerful stimulant. Infused in spirits, it makes an excellent wash in rheumatism.

GUM—CHERRY.

This gum, according to Dr. Stearns, is good in a thin, acrid state of the fluids; and where the mucus of the intestines is abraded; and therefore good in hoarseness; dysentery; diarrhœas; griping pains; hemorrhages; tickling coughs; salt; catarrhs; spitting of blood; heat of urine; and strangury.

HAZEL NUT BUSH.

The bark of this bush, mixed with an equal quantity of Wickopy bark, and boiled strong, makes an excellent wash in debility, and a low state of the blood.

It removes obstructions of the pores, and strengthens the system in general.

HEAD—BETONY.

The plant is corroborant and errhine. The roots are emetic and cathartic.

An infusion, or light decoction of the leaves, drank as a tea; or a saturated infusion in rectified spirits, is good in laxity and debility of the viscera, and disorders arising from thence.

HEDGE HOG.

This animal is found in various parts of America; and is held in high estimation by the Indians.

Its flesh they use for food; its oil for burns and scalds; and its quills serve as ornaments for their mockasins, peag, &c.

HELLEBORE—WHITE.

This is a powerful emetic; and so poisonous, that if eaten by swine or fowls, it proves immediately mortal.

The fresh roots, pulverized, and applied to the

bowels, promote the discharge of urine; and, applied to the regions of the liver, remove schirrhosities, and other affections, though of long standing.

HEMLOCK—GARDEN.

This plant is resolvent, discutient, narcotic, sedative and anodyne.

It is good in schirrhosities; scrofulous humors and ulcers; the chin cough; consumption; gleets; fluor albus; painful uterine discharges; venereal ulcers; epilepsies; convulsions; and to ease pain in open cancers; which it does more powerfully than opium. It procures sleep; eases pain; promotes sweat and urine; and, externally applied, discusses hard tumors.

The juice, put into a pewter dish, and dried away in the sun to the consistence of gum—then formed into pills, is a powerful anodyne, and helps when opiates fail; but taken in too large doses, it proves, like opium, highly detrimental.

HEMLOCK TREE.

This is a large tree, growing in many parts of America.

A decoction of the boughs has been used with success in rheumatic and sciatic complaints.

The pulverized bark is good in scurvy and canker.

A syrrup of the buds of hemlock and sweet fern, has been given for the destruction of worms; and a cataplasm of hemlock buds and Indian meal is an excellent remedy for scalds, burns, and freezes.

The Indians often cure the lumbago, by sweating the patient upon hemlock boughs, placed upon a flat stone, which has been heated in the fire, giving him decoctions of the boughs to drink, and covering him with a blanket.

HEMLOCK—GROUND.

The rheumatism may often be effectually cured by bathing the part affected with decoctions of this plant; and internally taken, it helps the St. Anthony's fire.

HEMP—COMMON.

The seeds are emollient and demulcent. A decoction of them in milk, or their watery emulsion, is esteemed good for a cough, and heat of urine.

HEMP—INDIAN.

This plant is anthelmintic, and a powerful diuretic.

The pulverized roots are an excellent remedy, given in molasses, for worms in children.

The expressed juice, mixed with an equal quantity of Holland gin, is almost a sovereign remedy in dropsies.

HEMP—AGRIMONY.

It grows wild by the sides of rivers and ditches. The leaves are aperient, laxative, anti-scorbutic and corroborant.

They are called good in the dropsy, jaundice,

cachexy, scurvy, and for strengthening the tone of the viscera.

Bœrhaave relates that the turf diggers in Holland use them in scurvy, swelling of the feet, and foul ulcers.

Decoctions of the root, in large doses, both vomit and purge. The Dutch use it in smaller doses, as an alternative and anti-scorbutic.

Dr. Lewis informs that it is useful in the beginning of dropsies, jaundice, intermitting fevers, and other disorders, arising from obstructions of the viscera, succeeding frequent relapses, and degenerating into acute, or a long continuance of chronic diseases.

HEN.

This is a domestic fowl, whose flesh is much used as food.

The eggs make a very nourishing and wholesome diet.

A broth, made of chickens, is very nourishing in fevers, and other disorders.

HENBANE—BLACK.

The common black henbane is a powerful narcotic, sedative, and anodyne.

It eases pain, procures sleep, helps the ophthalmia, and tooth-ache; resolves hard swellings; and is good in schirrhosities, open ulcers, palpitations of the heart, coughs, spasms, convulsions, epilepsy, melancholy, madness, hysterical complaints, and other nervous affections.

A cataplasm of the leaves and hog's lard, is very beneficial in glandular swellings and open ulcers. It is often a good substitute for opium; and may be proper when opiates affect the head. But, if taken in too large doses, it produces vertigo, head-ache, cholic pains, vomiting, a copious flow of urine, and sometimes a purging.

HOLLY HOCK.

This is chiefly cultivated as an ornament in gardens.

Its virtues are much the same as the common Mallows.*

---

* Vide Mallows.

HONESTY.

This plant is warming and diuretic.

It is cultivated in gardens. The stalk grows two or three feet high; the flowers are of a fleshy color: the leaves resemble those of a nettle, but larger.

HONEY

Is detergent, aperient, and expectorant.

Dr. Wallis calls it emollient, demulcent, and highly purgative.

It powerfully promotes expectoration; deterges and resolves rigidities in the primavia; temperates the acrimony of the humors; helps coughs, asthmas, disorders of the kidneys, and urinary passages; and the sore mouth and throat. It cleanses ulcers; purges moderately; and resists putrefaction.

It is used in gargarisms, decoctions and clysters.

It is hurtful to bilious, melancho'ic, hysterical, and hypochondriac habits.

HONEY-SUCKLE.

This plant is found in the swamps of Connecticut, and elsewhere.

It is deobstruent and anti-asthmatic.

Mixed with an equal quantity of air sponge, and taken in large doses, it is an excellent medicine in the asthma.

HOPS.

They are stimulant, balsamic, aperient and diuretic.

The flowers are powerfully anthelmintic. They are one of the most agreeable of the strong bitters.

Dr. Brooks informs that hops promote digestion; open obstructions; promote urine; loosen the belly; and are good in hypochondriac passion, scurvy, and other diseases of the skin, if taken in whey, or broth, as an alternative.

HOARHOUND—WHITE.

It is aperient and deobstruent.

It promotes the fluid secretions in general; and, taken freely, loosens the belly; helps humoral asthmas; coughs; yellow jaundice; cachexy; menstrual obstructions, and dropsy.

The juice, mixed with that of plantain, is good for the bite of a rattlesnake.

HOARHOUND—WATER.

This herb grows wild by the side of rivers and brooks.

It has the virtues of the white kind; but is much weaker.

HORSE RADISH.

The root is stimulant, expectorant, emetic, epispastic, and antiseptic.

It stimulates the solids; attenuates the fluids, and promotes the secretions, by extending its action through the whole habit to such a degree as to affect the minutest glands.

It promotes expectoration, sweat and urine;

excites an appetite in weak, relaxed stomachs, without heating too much.

It is good in palsies, rheumatisms, jaundice, cachexy, and dropsies; particularly those which follow intermitting fevers.

It is useful in some kinds of scurvy; and other chronic disorders, proceeding from a viscidity of the juices, or obstructions of the excretory ducts.

If the root is chewed, it excites spitting; and is good in want of taste, and a palsy of the tongue.

The juice is beneficial in dropsies, and gravel.

Poultices of the root, applied to the feet, are useful in fevers, unattended with delirium.

HOUND'S TONGUE.

The leaves of this plant, externally applied, heal contusions. The root also has been used in a gonorrhœa, and scrofulous complaints.

Dr. Fuller says he found a sirup of hound's tongue a second to a remedy against thin catarrhous humors, and a cough occasioned thereby.

Dr. Lewis informs, that decoctions of the root

have been used in catarrhs; coughs; diarrhœas; dysenteries and hemorrhages.

HOUSE LEEK.

The common house leek is cooling, emollient and laxative.

It quenches thirst; allays heat; and abates inflammations, tending to a gangrene.

They have also been called useful in bilious and burning fevers; for which purposes, the leaves must be steeped in water.

HYSSOP.

This plant has been esteemed attenuant, expecterant, and corroborant.

An infusion of the leaves with honey, is used in humoral asthmas; coughs; and other disorders of the breast, unaccompanied with inflammatory symptoms. It likewise promotes expectoration.

HYSSOP—HEDGE.

The leaves are emetic and cathartic: the roots have the same quality, but in a less degree.

Dr. Healde says it is anthelmintic, deobstruent, diuretic, and purgative.

The leaves have been used in dropsies; hip-gout; and the venereal disease, accompanied with tumors, ulcerations, and fluor albus. They excite sweat and urine; and promote salivation.

IPECACUANHA.

Of this root, there are four kinds:—the grey, the brown, the white, and the yellow. Of these kinds, the grey is the best.

It is a safe emetic, and possesses something of an astringent and antiseptic quality.

It is good in diarrhœas; dysenteries; leucorrhœs, and obstructions of long standing.

It promotes perspiration; suppresses alvine fluxes; and, given in small doses, checks menstrual hemorrhages; and is useful in coughs, pleurisies, peripneumonies, and spitting of blood.

IRON.

This is the only metal which seems to be friendly to the human system.

It is emmenagogic and corroborant.

It strengthens the stomach, and system in general; quickens the circulation; expands and rarifies the juices; raises the pulse, and renders the blood more florid; promotes deficient secretions; and restrains them, when immoderate.

But when the fibres are tense and rigid, and the circulation quick; or when there is any spasmodic contraction of the vessels, it is hurtful, with all its preparations.

ISINGLASS.

This is a solid, agglutinous substance, obtained from the air bladder of the sturgeon.

It is agglutinant, inspissant, and demulcent.

It is good in ulcerations of the lungs and fauces, for defluxions, the fluor albus, dysentery, and hemorrhages.

IVY—WILD, AMERICAN.

It runs on the ground, fences, and often climbs thirty or forty feet high, emitting a strong and disagreeable odour, which may be smelt at a considerable distance in a hot, clear day. The effluvia, floating in the currents of the circumambient air, not only strike the external parts of the human body, but are received into the lungs by inspiration, and thus laying the foundation for nausea, vomiting, intolerable itching, cutaneous eruptions, blindness, pain, fever, hard swellings, and ulcers.

To cure this, the oil of olives, given internally, and applied externally, is the best remedy I ever found. Some of the country people have given a saffron tea inwardly, and applied outwardly an ointment made by the marsh mallows in cream.

JACK BY THE HEDGE.

This plant grows in hedges, and shady, waste places.

It has a root something like an onion, which is a powerful stimulus, and good in inflammations of the eyes.

A poultice of the root, externally applied, is good in deafness.

JALAP.

This is a very celebrated cathartic.

It purges noxious and serous humors downwards; and is good in dropsy, anasarca, cachexy, and small pox, when there is not too much inflammation.

JUNIPER.

The berries are stimulant, stomachic, carminative, detergent, and diuretic.

The oil and spirit is also stimulant and diuretic. The wood is sudorific.

The watery extract is good in catarrhs, debilities of the stomach and intestines, and suppressions of urine in old age.

LADY'S SMOCK,
OR VALERIAN—AMERICAN.

This plant is anti-spasmodic, and anti-epileptic.

The flowers are good in spasmodic asthma, palsy, St. Vitus's dance. They also mend the appetite, and help the epilepsy.

The roots are stronger than the flowers. An infusion of them with an equal quantity of White Cohush and White Solomon's Seal is a safe and excellent medicine in time of pregnancy.

LAVENDER—SWEET.

This is warm, stimulant, and anodyne.

It is good in vertigo, menstrual obstructions, tremor in old age; and, in general, for all disorders of the head, nerves, and uterus.

It allays spasms; and, applied externally, in fomentations, is said to relieve paralytic limbs.

LEEKS, or WILD ONIONS.

They are a great anthelmintic and stimulant.

They are good in consumptions, gleets and fluor albus.

A cataplasm, applied to the soles of the feet, makes a revulsion from the head : and applied to the region of the throat, expels worms in children. They have, in many respects, the same virtues of the garlic.

LEECH, or BLOOD SUCKER.

They are useful for drawing blood, where the lancet cannot be used.

The best kind are those which live in clear, running streams, with sandy bottoms, and are of a grey color.

The expressed juice of the animals, sweetened with honey, has often cured the most obstinate whooping cough.

LEMON.

The juice is antalkaline, anti-scorbutic, and mildly refrigerant.

It is supposed to be the most potent remedy in the scurvy, belonging to the vegetable kingdom.

The peel is stimulant, and makes a good bitter.

LETTUCE—GARDEN.

The leaves are emollient, cooling, and anodyne.

Used as a salad, it mitigates the heat of the stomach, liver, and other viscera; relaxing their crisped and too greatly oscillating fibres, and restoring their functions, so as to procure sleep.

LETTUCE—WILD;
Called also LETTUCE LIVERWORT.

It is gently laxative, powerfully diuretic, and somewhat sudorific.

An extract of the juice, in small doses, is good in dropsies.

In those of long standing, and proceeding from obstructions of the viscera, half an ounce has been given in a day.

It agrees with the stomach; quenches thirst; opens the belly; purges off the urine, and promotes sweat.

Dr. Stearns says, that out of twenty-four patients who took this remedy in the dropsy, but one died.

LILY—POND, WHITE.

This is a great stomachic, and a slight carminative.

It is a great corrector of the internal viscera; and of a cleansing, suppurating nature.

It is good in coughs and consumptions; but the root should be pulverized and mixed with honey.

LILY OF THE VALLEY.

This is a good stomachic.

It is good in nervous affections, and catarrhous disorders, coughs, and peripneumonies. And roasted, and eaten freely, is good in cases of extreme debility.

LILY—MEADOW.

It is stomachic and anti-scorbutic.

It makes a good stomach bitter, and is good in scurvy.

LIME-WATER.

Lime water is prepared of calcined oyster shells, by putting half a pound into six quarts of boiling water.

This is diuretic; good in laxity and debility of the solids, and heat in the stomach.

LIQUORICE.

Of this valuable root, there is a species growing in many parts of New-England, which is equally as good as that brought from foreign climates, and far more congenial to our constitutions.

It grows wild on interval lands.

The roots are incrassative, emollient, demulcent, attenuant, expectorant, detergent and diuretic.

They abate thirst in dropsies, help defluxions of the breast, soften acrimonious humors, and prove gently detergent.

It is good in coughs, pleurisy, gravel, dysury, strangury, and intense pain.

It temperates salt, sharp humors; allays the heat of the blood; abates the acrimony of the humors; promotes urine; and thickens the sanguinary fluids, when too thin.

LOBELIA.

This is a safe emetic, and cathartic.

It helps the phthisic, and is good in canker.

With strong decoctions of this plant, well sweetened with sugar, the Indians effectually eradicate the venereal virus.

LIVERWORT—BROOK.

This is a species of moss, growing in small rivulets.

It is good in consumptions, whooping and common coughs, and affections of the liver.

LUNGWORT—COMMON.

This is found growing upon the north side of the soft maple in many parts of America.

It is good in coughs and defluxions of the lungs.

MADDER.

This plant is cultivated in gardens, and has a square jointed stalk, and a red root.

The subtile quality of which this root is possessed, renders it eminently useful as a resolvent and aperient.

It is good in obstructions of the urinary organs, uterus, and internal viscera. Likewise, in coagulations of the blood from contusions in the jaundice and dropsy.

MAIDEN HAIR.

This herb abounds with a neutral, saponaceous quality, approaching to nitre.

It is expectorant, mucilaginous and sub-astringent.

It is good in tickling coughs; hoarseness from acrid defluxions; in obstructions of the viscera; obstinate coughs, pleurisy, asthma, jaundice, disorders of the kidneys, and irregularities of the menses. It promotes the fluid secretions, and strengthens the tone of the fibres.

MACKIMUS—LOW.

This is a low shrub, growing upon upland. The leaf resembles in form the maple, and has a smell, upon bruising, like Dog Mackimus.

It is anti-venereal and obtunding.

It cleanses and purifies the blood and juices. It is good in venereal taints and most humors.

MAPLE—DWARF.

This is a small tree, growing in swampy land.

Decoctions of the bark and leaves purify the blood and juices; expel worms; and make a good wash in fever sores.

MARJORAM—SWEET.

This plant is aromatic. The leaves are errhine.

It is good in disorders of the head, and nervous uterine obstructions; humoral asthmas and catarrhs in old people. Also, for other disorders proceeding from a cold cause.

The oil, given internally, and applied externally, is good in palsies and nervous affections.

This oil, diluted with water, and applied to the nose of infants, when they are so stopped that they cannot suck, generally gives relief.

MARJORAM—WILD.

This plant grows wild on gravelly lands. It has firm, round stalks.

The virtues are much the same of thyme.

Infusions of the herb have been drunken as a tea in weakness of stomach, and disorders of the breast. They promote sweat, and the fluid secretions in general.

An essential oil is obtained by distillation, which is often used to mitigate pain in hollow teeth.

MALLOWS—COMMON.

This plant is emollient.

Decoctions of the leaves are good in dysenteries, heat and sharpness of the urine, and to obtund acrimonious humors.

MALLOWS—MARSH.

This is found upon the sea shore, between high and low water mark.

Every part of this valuable plant, more especially the root, yields a copious mucilage by boiling in water; and is frequently employed in emollient cataplasms; likewise in humid asthmas, hoarseness and dysenteries. Also, in nephritic and calculous complaints, it is frequently of eminent service; also, externally, for softening and maturating hard tumors; and was used by Dr. Fuller in the cure of some of those disorders, long before it was known to others.

It is likewise useful in phthisics.

MANDRAKE.

The root of this plant is discutient and cathartic, and good in obstructions of the bowels, and other viscera.

MANNA.

This is a mild and agreeable laxative, which may be safely taken by pregnant women, young children, and those laboring under debility. But it will not operate as a cathartic, unless taken in large doses.

It obtunds acrid humors; evacuates the offending matter; and is good in coughs, fevers, pleurisies, bilious complaints, gravel, and whooping cough.

MAPLE-SUGAR.

The sap, as it runs from the tree, is good in scurvy; and the sugar and molasses are good for coughs, and other disorders of the breast.

MARIGOLD.

This is stimulant, anodyne, and moderately styptic.

It has the virtues of the saffron, but in a less degree.

It is good in the measles. Decoctions of the herb or flowers drive them out.

MASTER WORT.

This is a great carminative, and anti-hysteric.

Dr. Fuller informs, that it is an excellent medicine in bilious and flatulent cholics.

It is useful in hysterics, and nervous complaints.

MAY WEED.

This herb is found growing in the highways in many parts of New-England.

Infusions of the herb have been given in recent colds, to promote sweat: but I have found that decoctions of Arsmart are far preferable.

MELILOT.

This plant is an emollient.

An ointment may be made by simmering this herb in fresh butter, or lard, which is of great use in foul ulcers and old sores.

MELON—WATER.

The fruit is a powerful diuretic; and is very cooling in hot, bilious constitutions.

The seeds, pulverized, and infused in Holland gin, make an excellent medicine in the dropsy.

MELON—MUSK.

These melons are raised in plenty in New-England; but they are not used in medicine.

They are not so wholesome as the water melon, but are apt to putrefy upon the stomach. They are nevertheless eaten freely by those to whom they are palatable.

MILK.

This is of great utility in medicine.

It is demulcent and nutricious, and therefore beneficial in consumptions, debility, scurvy, mineral and vegetable poisons, atrophy, gout, ephidrosis and strangury.

The milk of a woman is called better than any other kind for medical uses.

When this is taken in cases of extreme debility, it

should be sucked from the breast of a middle aged woman, of good habit, who lives temperately, and uses moderate exercise. The patient should suck about four hours after the woman has taken her meals. Milk drank immediately after it is taken from the cow, is likewise of great benefit in consumptions, and cases of debility, if it agrees with the patient: if not, it may be churned.

MILK WEED.

There is a variety of weeds of this name; but we would treat in particular, of the common, tall kind.

The juice of this is excellent in canker, and is said to cure warts.

MINERAL WATERS.

There are numbers of mineral springs in America, the most of which are in Saratoga and Ballstown, in the State of New-York.

Those of Saratoga are emetic, cathartic, and diuretic.

They are good in scrofulous and rheumatic affections; likewise, in venereal taints.

There is also a spring in Wilkes County, in Georgia, whose waters are excellent in the consumption, gout, rheumatism, scrofulous, scorbutic, and other maladies.

There are three springs in Wheelock, and another in Danville, Vermont, which promote digestion, and prove diuretic.

They cure the itch, and other cutaneous eruptions, and are of use in rheumatic complaints.

MINT—CAT.

This is emmenagogic, stimulant, and nervine.

It is good in recent colds; and an excellent application for fresh wounds, to stop bleeding.

It promotes the menses, and is good in jaundice, cough, and asthma.

MINT—HORSE.

This is emmenagogic, and powerfully stimulant.

Infusions of the herb are good in recent colds, nausea, and vomiting.

MINT—PEPPER.

This is likewise stimulant.

It restores the functions of the stomach; cures the hiccoughs, flatulent cholic, and hysterical depressions.

It promotes digestion, and stops vomiting.

MINT—SPEAR.

This herb is stimulant, stomachic, carminative and restringent.

Infusions of the leaves are good in weakness of stomach, loss of appetite, nausea, vomiting, gripes, cholic pains, lientery, immoderate fluxes, hysterical affections, and other debilities consequent upon delivery. It is, likewise, a provoker of venery.

MISTLETOE.

This makes a good bitter in jaundice, debility, and loss of appetite.

MOON WORT.

This weed grows upon burnt land, and is sometimes called *first growth fire-weed*.

An ointment may be made of this weed by simmering it in cream, which gives immediate relief in the hemorrhoids.

MOSS—CUP.

This species of moss is found in meadows, and is sometimes called meadow cups.

It is of a cooling nature. The leaves, applied to the part affected, cures the salt rheum.

MOTHER WORT.

This plant is deobstruent, laxative, diaphoretic,

diuretic, emmenagogic, anti-hysteric, anti-spasmodic, anthelmintic and corroborant.

Infusions of the leaves and tops open obstructions, relax the belly, promote insensible perspiration, urine, and the menses.

It is good in spasmodic and hysterical affections; convulsions; palpitations of the heart; to destroy worms, and strengthen the system.

MOUSE EAR.

This herb is cooling, and makes an excellent eye-water.

MUG WORT.

It is a mild emmenagogic, and anti-hysteric.

Taken in decoction and infusion, it removes pain from the head; promotes the menses, and allays hysterical spasms.

The expressed juice is useful in rheumatic and sciatic complaints.

MUSTARD.

The seed is stimulant, expectorant, emetic, purgative, aperient, and epispastic.

It stimulates the solids; attenuates the fluids; excites an appetite; promotes digestion; increases the fluid secretions; helps the palsey, rheumatism, scurvy, and milreek; loosens the belly; helps low fevers; and if given in whey, excites urine.

Applied in cataplasms, it relieves rheumatic pains, and paralytic affections.

Applied to the soles of the feet, it makes a revulsion from the head.

MUTTON SUET.

It is emollient, relaxing rigid parts, though harder in consistence than that of swine.

When mixed with bee's wax, it makes an excellent salve.

The oil, extracted, cures a diarrhœa in a short time. The dose for an adult, is one table spoonful.

NETTLE—STINGING.

This herb is a powerful styptic.

The juice, taken in small doses, is good in consumptions, and spitting blood.

Decoctions of the herb remove disorders of the bowels; and are good in diabetes and bloody urine.

The juice, snuffed up the nose, stops its bleeding; and stinging the parts affected, with nettles, helps the palsy, lethargy, and febrile stupidity.

NIGHT SHADE.

The leaves are cooling, and poisonous.

They are good in cancerous disorders, and foul ulcers, accompanied with pain.

The herb is good in scrofulous diseases, and obstinate pains in particular parts. The leaves, beat into a poultice, with white bread, or a salve made by simmering them in lard, abate inflammations in the eyes; ease the head ache; pains in the ears; help acrid defluxions, and inflammations of the venereal kind. But it is so poisonous, that none unacquainted with it, should venture upon its use.

NETTLE LIVERWORT.

This grows in bunches or clusters upon hard-wood land in various parts of New-England.

It is good in consumptions, coughs, and female weakness.

The herb should be gathered when in bloom.

OAK—WHITE.

The bark of this tree is a powerful styptic and astringent.

It is good in fluor albus, dysentery, and bloody fluxes; and a powder of the bark is excellent in open cancers.

OAK—RED.

Some have supposed the bark of this tree to

be as efficacious, in many disorders, as the Cort. Peru.

The following has been recommended as a cure for a cancer:

Boil the ashes of a bushel of red oak bark in three gallons of water, till two thirds are evaporated;—strain the liquor, and boil it again to the consistence of cream;—spread some of it on lint, and apply it to the cancerous sore. Renew the plaister every two hours. From four to twelve plaisters generally destroy the roots of the cancer, and work a complete cure.

OAK OF JERUSALEM.

This herb is cultivated in gardens.

It is emmenagogic, and a great deobstruent.

It stimulates the solids; attenuates the fluids; and is good in obstructions of the menses, urine, &c.

OLIVE.

They are the product of a tree growing in warmer climates.

The expressed oil is anthelmintic, and emollient.

It is a celebrated medicine in vegetable poisons, the bite of rattlesnakes, and many other disorders.

ONION.

This root is stimulant and diuretic.

It is good in gravel, strangury and scurvy; and applied to the soles of the feet, makes a revulsion from the head. The expressed juice of one onion is the proper dose, once in three hours.

They are much used as food, and make a very wholesome diet.

ORANGE.

The peel is aromatic, stimulant, stomachic and corroborant.

The juice is refrigerant, anti-septic and antiscorbutic.

The peel strengthens the stomach, and makes an excellent bitter.

OYSTER.

These make a very wholesome diet, either raw or cooked.

The calcined shells are good absorbents, and correct acidities in the primæ viæ.

PARSLEY.

This plant is refrigerant and diuretic.

It has been used in gravelly complaints; but I believe with very little success.

It is, however, cooling, and good in heat of urine.

PARSNIP.

The common garden parsnip is much used as food, and is highly nutritious.

It strengthens the system in general, and provokes venery.

It also sweetens acidities in the primæ viæ.

PARTRIDGE BERRY, or CHECKER-BERRY.

It is a powerful diuretic and absorbent.
The distilled liquor is useful in dropsy.

PEACH TREE.

The flowers are mildly laxative, and a good anthelmintic.

The leaves are stronger than the flowers.

The fruit is cooling and laxative.

An infusion of the leaves and flowers is given to children to purge the belly, and destroy worms.

PEARL ASHES.

The vegetable alkali is used in the form of lotions to correct acidities in the primæ viæ.

Infused in vinegar, it makes an excellent wash in fever-sores.

PENNY ROYAL.

This is stimulant, emmenagogic, expectorant, and anti-spasmodic.

It is good in spasms, whooping cough, obstruction of the menses, and to promote expectoration.

But its virtues are similar to those of horse mint.

PEPPER—BLACK.

This is stimulant and errhine.

It is good in cold disorders, to strengthen the lax fibres, and excite an oscillation; to increase the motion of the blood, assist digestion, and provoke venery.

But if used too freely, it disposes the viscera to inflammation, and proves very injurious in acrimonious humors.

PETTY MORREL.

This is astringent, emmenagogic, stomachic, and balsamic.

It removes obstructions; and the baked root is good in coughs.

The berries, infused in brandy, remove the gout from the stomach, when other remedies fail.

PINE.

The bark of the White Pine is healing and balsamic.

It strengthens the lax fibres, and is good in weakness of the lungs, and fluor albus.

PITCH.

This is an oily substance drawn from the pine. That of the white pine is good in plaisters to draw out refractory humors. Given in form of pills, with loaf sugar, it helps diabetes; and three pills of the same, taking one at a time, will generally cure the bleeding piles.

PLANTAIN—GREAT.

The leaves and seeds of this plant are mildly restringent and corroborant.

Both the leaves and seeds are good in phthisical complaints, spitting blood, alvine fluxes, hemorrhages, and dysentery. The juice, mixed with an equal quantity of the juice of white hoarhound, is an excellent antidote for the bite of a rattlesnake.

The bruised leaves are good in inflammations, fresh wounds, and old ulcers.

PLANTAIN—RATTLESNAKE.

This is a great stomachic, and purifier of the blood and juices.

Captain Carver informs that the Indians were so convinced of the virtues of this powerful antidote, that for a trifling bribe of spirituous liquor, they would permit a rattlesnake to drive his fangs into their flesh;—they then chew the leaves, and apply them immediately to the wound. They also swallow at the same time, the juice of the plant, which seldom fails of averting the dangerous symptoms.

PLANTAIN—TOAD, or LESSER PLANTAIN.

This is excellent in the cure of animal poisons.

If the juice be applied to the part affected, immediately, it cures the bite of the rattlesnake, the spider, the sting of the bee, &c.

Its virtues are similar to those of the Great Plantain.

POPLAR.

The bark of the black, red and white, is astringent, and anti-scorbutic.

It cures pleuritic pains in the side; and is good in scrofulous complaints, and makes a healing salve.

POPPY.

The heads of this plant produce the opium.

The whole herb is anodyne.

It eases pain, increases the circulation, and is good in cutaneous eruptions. The seeds destroy crickets.

POTATO.

This vegetable is easily raised and makes a very wholesome diet.

They may be eaten, either boiled, baked, roasted, or fried; but are the most wholesome roasted; and thus cooked and eaten with butter, they make a light and wholesome diet in fevers, whooping cough, &c.

A poultice, made of roasted potatoes, is good in burns.

QUICK SILVER.

This is found in a whitish mass, resembling brick poorly burnt.

It is volatilized by fire, and received by vapor, in glass vessels.

It has been employed in all disorders of the lungs, bilious fever, dysentery, yellow fever, inflammations, gout, rheumatism, jaundice, schirrhosities of the liver, canine madness, putrid sore throat, obstructions of the menses, intermitting fevers, &c. &c.

It has likewise been supposed to be the only remedy which will effectually eradicate the venereal virus; but I have often effected a complete cure with gladwin, or blue flag, when mercurials failed; and through a long course of practice I have generally found it more difficult to counteract the baneful effects of this poisonous mineral, than to combat the disorders for which it has been celebrated; and think I do not deviate from truth in saying that I have witnessed hundreds of the human species hurried out of time by using it. Notwithstanding, my opinion is, that in the itch and some other cutaneous eruptions, it might do good in the hands of those who understand it. But I have so often witnessed a contrary effect, that I should think I was endangering the lives of my fellow creatures were I to recommend it.

QUEEN OF THE MEADOW.

This is a tall plant, with smooth, brittle, reddish stalks, on which are clusters of white flowers, followed by crooked seeds set in a roundish head.

The plant is diuretic, aromatic, alexipharmic and carminative.

It is good in gravel, strangury, and uterine complaints.

RACOON.

The flesh of this animal is nourishing.

The oil is laxative, and good for burns, stiff joints, and rheumatic complaints.

RASPBERRY.

The berries are antalkaline, and cooling.

They quench thirst, abate heat, help diarrhœa, promote the natural secretions, and strengthen the viscera.

A decoction of the leaves and roots has cured the dysentery, when other remedies failed.

RADISH—GARDEN.

The roots are attenuant, and carminative.

All parts of the plant are anti-scorbutic.

The roots are frequently eaten with bread and butter; and are good in scurvies, obstructions of the glands, and other disorders, proceeding from viscid juices.

RATTLESNAKE.

The oil of this serpent is relaxing and penetrating; their gall anodyne. The oil will cure the quinsy in children almost instantaneously.

It softens contractions, rigidities, callosities, corns, &c.; and if dropped into the ear, it helps deafness.

ROSIN.

This is good in plaisters and unguents.*

RHEUMATISM WEED, or WINTER GREEN.

This herb is good in inflammations of the eyes, tooth-ache, and to relieve pain in the stomach.

It grows in dark, black timbered forests; is a low, evergreen vegetable; and is found in almost all parts of New-England.

RHUBARB—COMMON.

The root is cathartic and astringent.

It has been used in diarrhœas and dysenteries, and to carry off viscid bile, lodged in the bilious ducts.

ROSE BAY TREE.

This is found growing in the northern latitudes.

---

* Vide Turpentine.

A decoction of the bark is good in internal weakness.

ROSE—DAMASK.

This is powerfully nervine, cordial, aromatic, and gently laxative.

Drunken as a tea, it is good in head-ache. Taken in injection, it helps the piles; and is almost a sovereign remedy in the fluor albus. The other kinds have the same virtues, but in a less degree.

ROSEMARY.

This herb is stimulant and nervine.

It excites the oscillation of the nervous fibres, and restores their relaxed tone.

It strengthens the brain; helps the memory, dimness of sight, epilepsy, palsy, hysterical fits, menstrual suppressions and obstructions of the liver and spleen. It is of use in phlegmatic habits, and debilities of the nervous system.

ROSEMARY—MARSH.

This is an astringent and emetic.

It is likewise anthelmintic.

It is found growing upon the sea shore, between high and low water mark.

It is good in canker, and cures the canker-rash.

RUE—GARDEN.

This herb is anti-spasmodic, emmenagogic, attenuant, resolvent and deobstruent.

It is good in a languid circulation of the blood; for viscid phlegm, hysterical complaints, menstrual obstructions, and those of the excretory glands, as it promotes the fluid secretions in general.

It is, likewise, a powerful anthelmintic.

RUM.

This spirit, properly diluted with water, and drank with moderation, incrassates the thin fluids, strengthens the lax fibres, and warms the habit.

It is of use in external applications. But if drank to excess, it produces drunkenness, tremors, apoplexy, palsies, and a train of horrible symptoms, which often end in death.

RUSH.

This is a powerful diuretic.

It is good in gravel, strangury, and other uterine complaints.

SAFFRON—GARDEN.

It is highly cordial, aromatic, anti-spasmodic, attenuant, emmenegogic, and anodyne.

It exhilerates the spirits, and is good in disorders of the breast, female obstructions, hysterical depressions, spasms, palpitations of the heart, fainting fits, coughs, and asthma.

But if taken in too large doses, it occasions immoderate mirth, involuntary laughter, and such ill effects as follow the abuse of spirituous liquors.

SAGE.

It is cooling and astringent.

It is good in inward wounds and bruises, dissolving coagulated blood. An infusion of the leaves may be drank as a tea.

It is a good drink in time of pregnancy for those who are liable to abortion.

ST. JOHN'S WORT.

This herb is stomachic, deobstruent, and corroborant.

It is used for cleansing the first passages.

SALT—GLAUBER'S.

This is a mild and useful purgative; of a cooling nature; and if taken in small doses, proves diuretic and aperient.

It is useful in a variety of complaints, where cooling and gentle purgatives are necessary; but should be used mostly in the spring, on account of its cooling nature. Two portions answer all the purposes of once bleeding.

SANICLE.

This is stimulant, stomachic, deobstruent, emmenagogic, and vulnerary.

It helps recent colds, and promotes the natural secretions in general.

SARSAPARILLA.

This root is stimulant and emmenagogic.

It sweetens the blood and juices; is good in debilities, and should be taken in strong decoction.

SALT—EPSOM.

This is cathartic and gently diuretic.

It promotes sweat and urine, and is good in affections of the internal viscera, and should be used mostly in the spring of the year.

SASSAFRAS.

This is a great styptic; and according to Dr. Stearns, stimulant, aperient, diuretic, diaphoretic, and corroborant.

With it the Indians cure the most obstinate dysentery.

SCABIOUS.

It is good in consumptions, fluor albus, and strengthens the system in general.

It is said to cure the itch, and other cutaneous eruptions.

SHEEP.

Their flesh is very nourishing, and their fat is used in divers kinds of ointments.

A broth made of the meat is a very wholesome diet in dysenteries.

SKUNK.

The oil of this animal is good for scald head, and is used in making various kinds of ointments.

It is said that no putrid disorder will prevail within half a mile of the scent of this animal.

SNAKE ROOT.

It is one of the most potent of vegetables, and is stimulant, stomachic, deobstruent, and attenuant.

It is good in internal weakness.

SOAP.

The best hard soap is stimulant, cathartic, and deobstruent.

The black soap, particularly, is good for the itch and other cutaneous eruptions.

SOLOMON'S SEAL—WHITE.

This is a great stomachic, diuretic, corroborant, and deobstruent.

It incrassates the thin fluids, strengthens the stomach, and is good in time of pregnancy.

SORREL WOOD.

The leaves are anti-septic and astringent.

They allay heat, cool fevers, quench thirst, temperate the caustic bile, strengthen the heart, help scurvies, malignant and pestilential fevers, inflammatory and putrid disorders.

The juice, infused in good rum, and sweetened with sugar, is an Indian remedy for a cough.

SPERMACETI.

This is obtained from the head of the Spermaceti Whale.

It is emollient, deobstruent and stomachic.

It is good in pain, and erosions of the intestines.

SPIDER.

Of these animals there are various kinds in America.

The bites of the green and yellow kinds are so poisonous, that they sometimes prove fatal.

The juice of the plantain is a sovereign remedy, if applied in season.

SPLEEN WORT, or ROCK POLYPOD.

This is found growing in the fissures of rocks, and is of the brake kind.

It is stomachic and diuretic.

It is good in coughs, and pulmonary complaints.

It allays pain in the urinary passages, and gently carries off sand and gravel in the mean time, for which purpose, an infusion may be drunken as a tea.

STRAW-BERRY.

This fruit quenches thirst, abates heat, and strengthens the stomach.

The vine and leaves are astringent, diuretic, stomachic and corroborant.

SUCCORY.

Of this plant there are two kinds, the wild and tame, both of which may be used indifferently.

They are gently cathartic, aperient, attenuant, detergent and corroborant.

The juice is good in obstructions of the viscera, jaundice, cachexy, hectic fever, inflammations, consumptions, stubborn intermitting fevers, hypochondriac affections, cutaneous diseases, debility of the intestines, and other chronic disorders.

SUGAR—BROWN.

This is emollient, demulcent, and gently laxative.

It is good in coughs, hoarseness, consumptions, pleurisies, peripneumonies, scurvy, putrid fevers, and ulcers.

It sheaths acrimony, absterges ulcerations, and excites the urinary discharges.

Molasses, mixed with an equal quantity of boiling water has cured the dysentery, when other remedies failed.

SULPHUR

Is anthelmintic, diaphoretic, and purgative.

It destroys worms, promotes insensible perspiration, and loosens the belly.

It cures the itch, and other cutaneous eruptions, if internally given; and, externally applied, is good in coughs, asthma, gout, rheumatism and scorbutic complaints.

An ounce of sulphur, dissolved in a pint of rum or gin, is an excellent remedy in rheumatic pains and itch, and should be used both externally and internally.

SUMACH—COMMON.

The berries are powerfully styptic and astringent.

Strong decoctions of these berries, given in form of injection, restore the rectum to its natural functions.

An ointment, made by simmering the bark of the root of sumach in lard, will cure burns, without leaving a scar.

SUGAR CANDY.

This is prepared by boiling down the sugar to a thicker consistence than usual, and may be made either of white or brown sugar.

It is good in hoarseness, and tickling coughs, and if powdered and blowed into the eyes with a quill, is said to remove films from the sclerotic coat.

SUMMER SAVORY.

It is pungent, aromatic, diuretic, and emmenagogic.

It warms the habit, promotes urine and the menses, helps a cold stomach, and the moist asthma, by promoting an expectoration of thick viscid matter which stuffs up the lungs.

SUN DEW.

Dr. Cutler says that the whole of this plant is so acrimonious that it will corrode the skin; and that the juice, mixed with milk, and applied to the skin, removes freckles and sun-burns;—that the clear juice destroys warts and corns.

The plant is so injurious to cattle and sheep, on account of its acrimony, that it renders their viscera schirrhous. It is a very small plant, and may be found growing in meadows.

SUN FLOWER.

The seeds are stimulant and diuretic, and likewise emmenagogic.

They are good in coughs, and defluxions of the lungs.

SWALLOW WORT.

This plant is nervine, diuretic and emmenagogic.

It is good in hysteric fits, and has been used in catarrhal, cachetic and scrofulous disorders; to promote sweat and urine; cure the measles, plague, small pox, &c.

TAMARIND.

This is a good stomachic.

It is nourishing and good in weak stomachs; but if taken in large doses, it purges downwards.

TANSY—DOUBLE.

This herb is styptic, anthelmintic, and emmenagogic.

The juice has been used in the dropsy, cachexy, and fluor albus.

Applied in cataplasms to the bowels, it is good

in putrid fevers, and worn upon the necks of children, it expels worms.

And, indeed, the virtues of this herb are such that no family ought long to remain without it.

TANSY—SINGLE.

This is mildly astringent and corroborant.

It has been used in the fluor albus, diarrhœa, hemorrhages, and intermitting fever; for which purpose it may be taken in decoction.

TAR.

This is a thick, black, resinous juice, melted by fire, out of old pine and fir trees, and is good in plaisters.

A water is obtained by putting a pint of tar into a gallon of water, well warmed and stirred, then settled and poured off for use.

It is good in debilities in old age, and cancer humors.

TARTAR.

This is cooling, laxative, diuretic and cathartic. It opens obstructions of the viscera; is good in fevers, loss of appetite, &c.

THOROUGH WORT.

This herb is emetic, and cathartic. But the cathartic quality is the strongest. The expressed juice cleanses the stomach, and proves diuretic and powerfully emetic and cathartic.

THISTLE—BULL.

This grows in highways and waste places, and is the largest kind of thistle.

It is detergent, and will cure the quinsy, when other medicines fail.

THORN BUSH.

The bark of this bush is astringent.

It is good in hysterics, cholics; and in decoction, it relieves pain in the bowels generally.

THYME—MOTHER.

This is a warm and pungent herb.

It is good in teeth-ache, and rheumatic complaints.

TIN.

A powder is prepared from tin, which is powerfully anthelmintic.

It is prepared in the following manner, viz:

Melt six pounds of tin in an earthen vessel, and stir it with an iron rod, till a powder floats upon the surface. Take off the powder, and when cold, pass it through a sieve.

This is given to destroy worms, particularly the tape worm.

TOBACCO.

This is a violent emetic and cathartic. It is also narcotic.

This is principally used for smoking and chewing, and is good in the phthisic and many disorders, but is generally injurious to the slender and consumptive.

TORMENTIL;

Called also SECOND GROWTH FIREWEED, BUTCHER'S BROOM, &c.

It grows upon burnt land, and is very troublesome among grain, where burnt land is sowed the second year.

It is a powerful astringent, and a sure and efficacious medicine in diarrhœas, dysenteries, and hemorrhages; but must be used with caution, lest the flux be stopped too soon.

TURNIP.

I shall speak of two kinds—the English and the French.

The French turnip is diuretic, expectorant, and discutient.

The juice, sweetened with honey or sugar, is good for coughs, and disorders of the breast.

Cataplasms of the grated root discuss dropsical swellings. The English have the same virtues, but are weaker.

VERVAIN.

This weed grows in highways, and has blue flowers upon the top, which resembles in shape the top of a corn stalk.

It is emetic, emmenagogic, and deobstruent.

It removes uterine obstructions, and, baked in a new earthen vessel, is an excellent remedy in consumptions.

VINEGAR.

It promotes expectoration, neutralizes alkaline

substances in the primæ viæ, cools inflammatory disorders, promotes sweat, and resists putrefaction.

It is good, both internally and externally, in all kinds of inflammatory, bilious, pestilential, malignant, and putrid disorders; for weakness, syncope, vomiting, lethargy, hypochondriac and hysterical affections, hydrophobia, and the ill effects of opium, hemlock, henbane, deadly night shade, &c.

But too much of it coagulates the chyle, produces leanness, atrophy, tubercles in the lungs, and consumptions.

VIOLET.

Of these there are several kinds; but those of which I would speak more particularly are the white and yellow.

They make a good common drink in strangury and gravelly complaints.

WALNUT—BLACK.

The bark is emetic, and cathartic, and is good in cold, languid habits.

A gill of the ashes of the bark of walnut, steeped in cider, and a gill of the liquor drank in the morning, fasting, is good in the jaundice.

WATER CRESS.

This herb is acrid, aperient, and cooling.

It is good in fevers, scurvy, and other febrile complaints.

WATER DOCK.

It grows about rivers, and other watery grounds, and has leaves two or three feet long.

The leaves are laxative, and anti-scorbutic. The roots are excellent in the scurvy, and cutaneous disorders, if internally given and externally applied in ointments, cataplasms, lotions, and fomentations. A strong decoction of the bark stops the eating of ulcers in the mouth and tonsels, and spongy gums.

WHEY.

This is cooling, diluent and aperient.

It promotes the natural secretions, opens the body, cleanses the first passages, prevents constipation, proves diuretic, and is good in pregnancy, rheumatism, bilious, burning and malignant fevers, ebullitions of the blood, tedious chronic complaints, heat of the liver and kidneys, scorching and melancholic humors, exciting wandering heats.

WILLOW—COMMON.

It is diuretic, deobstruent, anthelmintic, and antivenereal.

It is good in scorbutic and venereal complaints.

WINE.

Good wine stimulates the solids, cheers the spirits, warms the habit, promotes perspiration, renders the vessels full and turgid, raises the pulse, and quickens the circulation. Claret, Madeira, and Port are used in fevers of a typhus kind with success, when the stomach is weak, rejects all food, and the wine agrees with the patient. It is good in languors, debility, and a low state of fevers: also, for resisting putrefaction.

WINTER'S BARK.

This bark is the product of one of the largest forest trees on Terra del Fuego.

The bark is astringent, deobstruent, and antiscorbutic. It is good in scurvy and dropsy, and for intermitting and remitting fevers.

WINTER GREEN.

This is excellent in the rheumatism, and a good stomachic.

It cures spongy gums, and fastens loose teeth.

It is said that this root chewed six weeks every spring by young people, totally prevents the toothache.

WORM WOOD.

This is stomachic, discutient, corroborant, stimulant, antiseptic, and anthelmintic.

The essential oil is anti-spasmodic and anthelmintic.

Wormwood heats the body, attenuates viscid humors, increases the oscillation of the fibres, and promotes perspiration.

It opens obstructions, excites an appetite, strengthens the stomach, stops looseness, appeases the wind cholic, and restores the debilitated functions.

It is good in the jaundice, dropsy, green sickness, cachexy, agues, and to destroy worms.

It has also been employed externally in discutient and anti-septic fomentations.

The essential oil, diluted with brandy, is good in tertian agues, and if applied to the belly, and taken internally, kills worms. But is injurious in inflammations, and a crispiness and tensity of the fibres, and also to the eye-sight.

YARROW.

It is cooling, astringent and styptic. It is good in hemorrhages, dysenteries and diarrhœas; and if used as a constant drink for three days, it prevents the nose-bleed for a year.

END OF THE FIRST VOLUME.

THE

AMERICAN BOTANIST

AND

FAMILY PHYSICIAN.

TWO VOLUMES IN ONE.

VOL. II.

By John Monroe.

COMPILED BY SILAS GASKILL.

WHEELOCK, (VT.) PUBLISHED BY JONATHAN MORRISON.
Danville—Eben'r. Eaton, Printer.
1824.

THE AMERICAN BOTANIST
AND
FAMILY PHYSICIAN.

VOL. II.

INTERMITTING FEVER.

IN the beginning of this disorder,
Take two pounds of common Arsmart,
Two pounds of White Ash bark,
Two handfuls of Jerusalem Oak,
and One pound of Horse Radish.

Put these together into an iron kettle, and after adding one pailful of water, boil it over a gentle fire, until reduced to one quart.

To the liquor add one quart of Holland gin, and sweeten it with loaf sugar. Of this liquor let the patient drink three or four glasses in a day, giving freely strong infusions of Arsmart in the mean time.

PUTRID FEVER.

In the beginning of this disorder, it will be necessary to cleanse the first passages. For this purpose an emetic of lobelia may be given, and afterwards one portion of Glauber's salts. After this, continue to give portions of the Universal Pill every night through the disorder, for the purpose of keeping the bowels gently open.

Infusions of equal quantities of cool wort, and black maiden hair, should be drank freely. Likewise soda or white lye should be given freely.

Take one handful of bark from the north side of the Black Ash.
>One handful of the bark of Wild Cherry.
>One handful of Sweet Poplar bark.
>One handful of Dog Mackimus bark,

and One handful of Sweet Elder bark.

Boil these together into a sirup of one quart. Add to it one quart of wine, and continue to give six glasses in a day of this liquor, or as the patient can bear through the disorder.

It will likewise be proper to apply cataplasms of horse radish root to the soles of the feet.

I have known patients in the last stage of this disorder completely cured by drinking freely of water, or rum and water.

Powders of the bark of dog mackimus answer all the purposes for which the Jesuits bark is intended, and should be given once in six hours through the disorder.

SPOTTED, or SCARLET FEVER.

In the beginning of this disorder, let an emetic of lobelia be administered in order to throw off the bile from the stomach; and after this, sweat profusely with hemlock boughs.

For a common drink, take equal parts of Sarsaparilla, Burdock, and Sweet Elder. Boil these together, and let the patient drink freely, until he is perfectly recovered, which will generally be in a few days. It will likewise be proper to administer a portion of the universal pill once in two or three days.

PLEURISY.

On the first attack of this disorder, it will be necessary for the patient to lose a little blood. After this, sweat freely with hemlock, and let the patient drink constantly decoctions of the bark of the 'Conead or Black Poplar. If this cannot be had, the White Poplar will answer much the same purpose.

Cataplasms of mustard seed, or the root of Horse Radish, should likewise be applied to the soles of the feet.

INFLAMMATION OF THE BOWELS,
and other viscera.

In the beginning of this disorder, take good vinegar, and add to it as much pearlash as it will dissolve, and with it bathe the part affected once in an hour; or take the berries of sumach, bruise and put them into hot water; then add vinegar, and thicken with wheat bran. Apply this cataplasm to the part affected.

If this should not give relief, take the roots of

common Hellebore, bruise them to a poultice, and lay this upon the part diseased. A poultice may likewise be made of yeast and barley malt, which is often of great service. Let this be applied to the part affected, and changed as often as necessary.

INFLAMMATION OF THE BRAIN.

When the person is attacked by this alarming disorder, take strong decoctions of hops; add an equal quantity of spirits, and with it bathe the head continually.

For a common drink, take equal quantities of Burdock and Sarsaparilla, and boil together strong, and let the patient drink freely of the liquor.

INFLAMMATION OF THE EYES.

Take the garden Chamomile, boil it in new milk, strain and add to the liquor, an equal quantity of West India rum, and sweeten it with loaf sugar.

With this liquor, bathe the temples and eyes

three or four times in a day, until they are completely cured.

This is an excellent eye-water in almost any kind of sore eyes.

BILIOUS CHOLIC.

This seems to be a kind of hereditary distemper, to which some constitutions are particularly subject.

When the person is attacked with it, give an injection of Thorough Wort, boiled strong, and let the patient drink freely of the same herb.

If this should not effect a cure, give an injection of tobacco leaves, boiled strong, and afterwards a sirup of the bark of thorn, which will seldom fail of effecting a cure.

DIABETES.

Strong decoctions of the Stinging Nettle, drank freely, will, in most cases, effectually cure.

The patient should take likewise one or two

portions of the universal pill, and afterwards decoctions of the bark of thorn.

If this should not have the effect desired, take the gum of the spruce tree; infuse this in spirits, and let the patient drink moderately of the same. This I have never known to fail.

DYSENTERY.

In the beginning of this disorder, let the patient take of the Cream of Tartar, one tea spoonful at a time four times in a day, continuing it for two days. This will operate as a cathartic, and answer all the purposes of an emetic. The patient should drink all the while strong decoctions of Sweet Agrimony infused in an equal quantity of brandy, and sweetened with loaf sugar, one glass at a time, as often as he can bear.

GRAVEL, or STONE.

To cure this distressing disorder,
Take One handful of Lobelia,

One handful of Violets,
One handful of Chamomile,
and One handful of Clivers.

Steep these together, and reduce the liquor to one quart. Add to it one pint white lye, and one quart Holland gin.

Of this liquor let the patient drink freely six or seven times in a day, and drink likewise a glass of onion juice every night for nine nights.

This cures the gravel almost infallibly, which it does by neutralizing and dissolving the stone. It will continue to come away from the patient for twenty-four hours in the form of fine sand.

JAUNDICE.

It will be highly necessary in the beginning of this disorder, to throw off the bile from the stomach, and cleanse the first passages.

For this purpose strong decoctions of Thorough Wort should be given. If this should not operate as an emetic, let the patient take of the expressed juice of the herb two thirds of a tea-cup full.

After this, infusions of the Ground Ivy should be drank freely as a common drink, and one glass of the expressed juice of Celendyne, three times in a day.

If this course be pursued, the patient will seldom be disappointed of a cure.

WHOOPING COUGH.

Take equal parts of Lobelia, Hyssop, and the berries of Sumach.

Boil these together strong, and sweeten the liquor with loaf sugar.

Give this preparation in form of drops, to the quantity of ten at a time, once in three hours, and increase the dose, as the patient can bear.

The juice of onions, or leeks, drank freely, will be also proper, and give great relief.

If this should not effect a cure, take a handful of Brook Liverwort, and steep it in a pint of the urine of a healthy person; then strain off the liquor, and sweeten it with honey or molasses.

The dose of this is a tea-spoonful once in half

an hour, for a child under three years old. For a child over three and under six, it should be double that quantity, and so on in proportion to the age.

MEASLES.

In this disorder the greatest care ought always to be observed.

The patient should not expose himself to take cold by wearing damp clothes, wetting his feet, or appearing in the evening air; but should continually drink something of a stimulating nature, such as infusions of the garden Marigold, &c.

CANKER-RASH.

This fatal disorder, which has so often spread terror through New-England, if properly treated, will seldom prove mortal.

In the first stage of this disorder, let the patient take of the infusion of Lobelia, until it proves emetic. Afterwards take one ounce of pulverized

Bloodroot, half a pint of vinegar, and two ounces of honey. After having mixed these properly together, let the patient take of the mixture a teaspoonful once in half an hour.

It will likewise be proper to let the patient drink of soda, dissolved in water, once an hour, as long as there is any appearance of canker.

DROPSY.

Take equal parts of the juice of India Hemp-roots, and Holland gin, and let the patient drink of this mixture one glass at a time, four or five times in a day, drinking all the while, infusions of the roots of Dwarf Elder, and of the distilled liquor of cuckoo ash, one pint in a day.

The most proper diet in this disorder will be fresh meat, roasted, and hard biscuit.

PHTHISIC AND ASTHMA.

Take the Consumption Dock, and boil strong.

Take of this decoction one quart. Add to it one pint of Holland gin, and let the patient drink freely of this mixture through the disorder; continuing to take the universal pill every night, one portion at a time, or enough to operate.

This will generally carry off the disorder, where it is curable.

BLEEDING AT THE LUNGS.

Take one quart of good brandy; bruise and put into it one half pound of the inside of Buckhorn Brake root. After it has stood a short time, it coagulates, and appears like the white of an egg.

Let the patient take of this liquid, one glass at a time, four times in a day, or a table spoonful once in twenty minutes.

This I can pronounce almost an infallible cure, if duly persisted in.

It is likewise good in a cough, and weakness of the stomach.

But if this should not effect a cure, the patient may drink of the expressed juice of Tormentil, one half glass in a day, or take in substance a teaspoonful of the pulverized root of Bistort.

CONSUMPTION COUGH.

Take two handfuls of Maple Lungwort,
    One and an half handful of White Oak Liverwort,
    One handful of Brook Liverwort,
    One handful of Hyssop,
    One handful of Licorice,
    One handful of Hoarhound,
and One handful of Penny Royal.

Boil these together in one pailful of water, until the liquor is reduced to two quarts. Add to it one pint of rum, and one pint of molasses.

Let the patient take of this liquor six or seven glasses in a day.

If, after this, the cough should continue, a sirup may be used of the following description:
Take One half pound White Solomon's Seal roots,
    Two pounds of Hog Brake roots,

Four ounces of Arsmart,
One half peck of Alder tags.

Boil these together in one pailful of water, till the liquor is reduced to one quart. Add to it one pint of West India Rum, and sweeten it with sugar.

Of this it will be proper to take three glasses in a day.

If this should not have the desired effect, and the cough should still continue, take one pint of Wood Sorrel juice, and add to it one pint of New-England Rum, and sweeten it with loaf sugar, and let the patient take of this liquor five or six glasses in a day.

CONSUMPTION.

To cure this alarming disorder,
Take Four ounces of Sweet Elder bark,
Four ounces of Dog Mackimus,
Two large Wake Robins,
One handful of Chamomile,
One handful of Brook Lime,
Four ounces of White Ash bark,

One pound of Celendyne,
One pound of Nettle roots,
and Two pounds of Ground Ivy.

Boil these together in two pailfuls of water, throw out the herbs, and reduce the liquor to two quarts. Add to it two quarts of Holland gin, and sweeten it with Maple sugar to the patient's liking.

Of this liquor, let the patient drink two thirds of a glass six times a day.

If, notwithstanding, the disorder should be attended with any considerable degree of cough, it will be necessary to promote the expectoration, and check the cough. For this purpose, see Consumption Cough.

PALSY.

Upon the first attack of this disorder, the patient should take the roots and tops of the stinging Nettle in strong decoction, and continue to whip the part affected with the green tops of the same herb.

This method of treatment, if duly persisted in, will seldom fail of working a cure.

EPILEPSY.

Take the American Valerian; boil it strong, and let the patient drink freely of the decoction, or take the pulverized root of the same herb, in form of powders three times in a day, to the quantity of a tea-spoonful at a time.

If the above medicine should not effect a cure, let the patient take of the flour of tin two grains in a day for three days successively; after which give decoctions of the tags of Alder.

The last mentioned medicine, when the disorder proceeds from the tape worm, will effectually cure, by destroying the animal.

WORMS.

Take One quart of Hemlock buds,
  Two pounds of Sweet Fern roots and tops,
and Two pounds of Alder tags or tops.

Boil these together in one pailful of water until you reduce it to one quart. Sweeten it with loaf sugar, and let the patient drink of it three glasses in a day.

If this should not have the desired effect, take equal quantities of Sweet Fern roots, and the bark of White Walnut roots; dry and pound them, mix them with West India molasses, and let the patient take, if an adult, one tea-spoonful three times in a day; if a child five years of age one half that quantity. For a child two years old, take strong decoctions of Tamerack bark, infused in brandy, and sweetened with loaf sugar; into this put the powder of Blood root and Wild Turnip, and give one tea-spoonful at a time.

HEART BURN.

Many medicines are good for this disorder, such as magnesia, chalk, &c. But the Indian method for curing this disorder, is, to swallow a fish-worm alive. This will effectually cure it, and prevent it from ever returning.

QUINSY.

This distressing disorder is principally confined

to children, although it seems to be a species of asthma.

The oil of the rattlesnake is a sovereign remedy in this disorder, and should be given internally.

If this cannot be had, let the juice of the common bull Thistle be given, which will often cure, when other remedies fail.

RICKETS.

Let the child be put into a cold bath three mornings successively; then miss three mornings, and proceed in this way until the child has been bathed nine mornings. After taking it out of the bath each time, wrap it in a blanket, and lay it in a warm bed.

Fill a cradle with the hog brakes, and let the child sleep constantly upon them, giving it decoctions of the root to drink.

This mode of treatment will seldom fail of effecting a complete cure.

MUMPS.

In this disorder the patient should not expose himself to take cold in the damp air, or by wetting his feet, but should continually have recourse to stimulating spirits, and bathe the swelling with the same.

If the patient should swell downwards, take white beans, pound them fine, and make a poultice of them in milk and water, and apply to the swelling.

If this should not check the swelling, take the garden Chamomile and simmer it in milk, and with the liquor bathe the part affected, and drink infusions of the herb.

A wash made of the roots and tops of Bitter-Sweet is likewise an excellent remedy, and should be taken internally, and applied externally.

SMALL POX.

This disorder, which frequently appears in seaport towns, and spreads terror and dismay among the neighboring inhabitants, if properly treated, would seldom prove mortal.

When the patient is first attacked, he should have recourse immediately to strong decoctions of Gladwin, or Blue Flag. Milk and water is likewise a very proper drink. He should be kept in a cool situation, and receive, as much as possible, the benefit of the fresh air.

If the pustules should not appear before he begins to swell, he should drink freely of milk punch. This will generally cause them to appear.

CATARRH IN THE HEAD.

Take the Ground Ivy, when it is in bloom; dry it and make a powder, which use constantly for snuff. Take Four ounces of the roots of Bitter-Sweet,
      One pound of Celendyne;
      One pound of Dog Mackimus bark,
and   One pound of Ground Ivy.

Boil these together in one and a half pailfuls of water, until the liquor is reduced to one quart. Add to it one quart of Holland gin. Of this mixture take four glasses in a day before eating.

If a sore collect in the ear, take the heart of a roasted onion, and insert into the ear, and apply a poultice of the same to the outside of it; then smoke the nostrils with the bark of Dog Mackimus.

LOCK JAW.

On the first appearance of this disorder, pour down as much salt and water as possible. This alone will often entirely cure.

If the jaws continue set, or so closely drawn together that nothing can be taken, take two ounces of good tobacco, and steep strong, and give it in form of injection.

This repeated two or three times will generally give relief. Afterwards it will be necessary to give strengthening sirups.

VIRULENT GONORRHŒA.

This is the name applied to the venereal disorder in its first stage.

On the first appearance of this disorder, the patient should immediately have recourse to strong decoctions of Gladwin or blue flag roots, which should be drank freely; and for a common drink, take decoctions of Lobelia and Dog Mackimus as often as can be borne.

This method of treatment, if persisted in, will seldom fail of effecting a cure, when even mercurials fail.

HYDROPHOBIA,
AND BITE OF A RATTLESNAKE.

When the person is attacked with either of these terrible disorders, take strong decoctions of Lobelia, both internally, and apply externally to the part affected; or if the green herb can be had, the clear juice should be applied to the part affected, and he should drink freely of the decoction.

If this be resorted to in season, it will cure immediately.

The juice of the common Plantain is an excellent medicine, and should be given internally, and applied externally.

PILES, or HEMORRHOIDS.

In the beginning of this distressing disorder, make an ointment of Celendyne and Moonwort in fresh butter. With this anoint the part; at the same time give a decoction of the berries of Sumach, in the form of an injection. This will prove a powerful remedy. For a common drink,
Take Two pounds of Celendyne,
    Two pounds of Cedar boughs,
and Two handfuls of Coolwort.

Of these make a decoction, and let the patient drink freely.

If the injection of Sumach should not have the desired effect, give an injection of Damask Roses.

This mode of treatment will seldom fail of effecting a complete cure.

It effectually cured Dr. Meigs, late of Lyndon, Vermont, after he was considered incurable.

CRAMPS.

When attacked by this disorder, let sulphur be applied to the part affected.

- If an internal spasm, let the patient take sulphur, infused in spirits.

GOUT.

Take strong decoctions of the garden Pepper, and add to it an equal quantity of rum. With this liquor bathe the part affected as warm as it can be borne.

Take one large Bloodroot, pulverize and infuse it into a quart of spirits. Of this liquor let the patient take a table spoonful once in twenty minutes, until it makes him sick at the stomach. After this, take smaller quantities, until the sickness abates; then increase to a spoonful, until it sickens, and proceed in this way until the quart is expended.

RHEUMATISM.

[Bathe] the part affected with the Red or Garden Pepper, steeped strong in spirits, or make a plaister in the following manner:

Take Cedar boughs, Beach bark, and Comfrey roots of each the like quantity. Boil these together until the strength is boiled out; throw them out and boil the liquor to the consistence of a plaister. Apply this to the part affected, and it will generally give relief in a short time.

The patient should likewise take a portion of the universal pills.

A plaister of the balsam Racasari will often give great relief.

The patient should give himself to gentle exercise, such as riding on horseback, or in a carriage.

SPRAINS.

Take One handful of the bark of the Hazle,
    One pint of Vinegar,
and   One gill of Salt.

Simmer these well together, and with the liquor

wash the part affected, which will generally cure in a few days: But if it should not prove effectual,

Take One quart of Beef brine,

and One handful of Wormwood.

Simmer these together, and continue to scum the liquor until the particles have done rising. With this liquor bathe the part affected, and bind on the leaves of Wormwood, or Wormwood simmered in chamberlye may be applied; but where there is no inflammation of the part the balsam Racasari is the best application that I have ever found.

If, after applying the above medicines, the limb should continue weak, boil Alder bark in chamberlye, and with this bathe the part affected three times in a day.

CALLOUS.

To cure this affection, make a soap of Liver oil and the ashes of White Ash; throw into it Yellow Lily roots, as long as it will eat them up. Apply this to the part affected, which will soften and remove the callous.

SALT RHEUM.

Take the berries of Garget or Stoke, and make an ointment by simmering them in fresh butter or lard. With this anoint the part affected frequently, which will seldom fail of curing.

For a common drink, take, freely, infusions of Lettuce Liverwort.

ST. ANTHONY'S FIRE.

Take equal quantities of Wild Lettuce, Burdock and Sweet Elder bark, and boil them together. Let the patient drink freely of this liquor.

Take, likewise, Ground Hemlock and Bitter-Sweet, and boil them together strong, and bathe the whole body with this decoction.

SCALD HEAD.

Take one pint of Tar, and put it into a gallon of water; warm it well, and stir well together. Let it settle, and pour it off for use. With this wash the head of the child frequently, or shave off the hair, and let it wear a tarred cap. To cleanse the blood,

Take One peck of Sarsaparilla roots,
    Half a peck of Burdock roots,
and One handful of Dog Mackimus bark.

Boil these together, and let the child drink freely of the liquor.

BURN, OR SCALD.

Take the bark or berries of Sumach; boil in milk and water, and make a poultice by stirring into it Indian meal. Apply this to the part affected, and repeat it as often as is necessary.

This will effectually restore the muscles, and heal the sore, without leaving any scar.

If this cannot be had, take Basswood sprouts and scrape off the bark. Boil this in milk and water, and thicken it with Indian meal to the consistence of a poultice, and apply it to the part affected for three days, which will generally give relief.

CANCER, or HOLDFAST.

In this alarming disease, no individual medicine has yet been found, which, in all cases, has proved a sure and infallible antidote. Yet there are many which have often effected a complete cure. Of these I shall proceed to name the principal:

Take the juice of the berries of Garget; put it into a new pewter dish, and dry it away in the sun to the consistence of salve; spread this upon lint, and apply it to the sore four times in a day.

If this should not prove effectual, the juice of Wood Sorrel, or the juice of White Ash, which issues out of the stick, while burning, may be applied seven times in a day. These have cured many. Or,

Take the juice of Wood Sorrel and yellow Dock roots: Put these into a pewter vessel, and dry in the sun to the consistence of an ointment. Apply this to the cancerous sore seven times in a day.

If the patient should not experience relief from the foregoing medicines,

Take Garden Hemlock, and boil to the consistence of ointment. Apply this to the part affected, and make pills of the same by rolling them in the ashes of the same herb as large as a kernel of wheat, and let the patient swallow one of these pills in a day. This has cured many, but it is so very poisonous that great caution should be used in taking it internally.

The juice of Celendyne has often cured.

But for occult cancers, take one bushel of Red Oak bark, and boil it strong: then take out the bark and boil the liquor to the consistence of salve. Spread this upon dry lint, and apply it to the part affected, which will often draw a cancer completely out in nine days. The fœtid liquor contained in the bag of the skunk will likewise often cure in a short time.

ROSE CANCER.

Take one bushel of Tobacco stalks, and burn

them in a kettle to ashes. Leach the ashes in the urine of a healthy person. Add to this lye one quart of white lye, made of the ashes of black Ash, and boil the lyes together to the consistence of a plaister. Apply this seven times in a day.

This has often cured, when the patient was considered incurable.

The buds of the Balm of Gilead, pounded, and laid on, are excellent, and will often cure.

It will likewise be necessary to cleanse the blood, and eradicate effectually from the system this poisonous humor. For this purpose,
Take Two handfuls of Noble Liverwort,
    Two pounds of Sarsaparilla roots,
    One pound of Dog Mackimus bark,
and Four pounds of Sweet Fern roots and tops.

Boil these together strong. Add to it gin, and sweeten it with maple sugar. Let the patient drink of the liquor four glasses in a day. Or,
Take One handful of Wild Succory,
    One handful of Celendyne,
    One handful of Sweet Elder,
and One handful of Cancer roots.

Of these make a decoction; sweeten the same, and drink of it freely

KING'S EVIL.

Take the roots of Hellebore, pound and wet them with vinegar, and apply this poultice to the part affected.

For a common drink, take equal quantities of Wild Lettuce and Noble Liverwort; infuse them in water, and let the patient drink freely.

Codfish skins applied to the part affected, will often cure.

FEVER SORE.

Take equal quantities of the bark of Dog Mackimus, Dwarf Maple, and Low Mackimus. Boil these strong together, and add one third West India molasses. With this wash, syringe and cleanse the sore three or more times in a day.

Take vinegar, and add as much pearlash to it as it will dissolve. With this continue to wash the sore three times in a day.

The patient should likewise drink freely decoctions of the Yellow Dock, infused in spirits.

WHITE SWELLING.

Let the part affected be bathed frequently in cold water.

Take the common Honey Bees, and infuse them in spirits. Apply this spirit to the part affected immediately after bathing. If this should not have the desired effect, it will be necessary to blister the part thoroughly. The best application for this purpose is the flowers of Crowsfoot.

TO MAKE THE UNIVERSAL PILL CATHOLICON,

Take One armful of Thorough Wort,
One peck of White Ash bark,
One armful of Celendyne,
Half bushel of Butternut bark,
Four pounds of Sweet Elder bark,
Four pounds of Dog Mackimus,
Six pounds of Sarsaparilla,
Four large Wake Robins,
One pound of Blood Root,
Two pounds of Baisam bark,

Two handfuls of Gill go by the ground,
One peck of Burdock roots,
Two armfuls of Arsmart,
One peck of Cuckoo Ash,
One pound of Snake root,
Two pounds of Spruce bark,
One peck of Tamerack bark,

Boil these seperately, until the strength is out; then throw out the herbs and barks; settle the liquors, and boil them together to the consistence of tar.

Take White Ash bark, and burn it to ashes. With the above mentioned gum make pills by rolling it in the ashes as large as a pea. The proper dose of these is from seven to twelve for an adult.

These give relief in pain in the stomach, jaundice, and bilious complaints; all kinds of inflammatory and chronical disorders, and a safe and efficacious remedy in all cases where physic is necessary.

TO MAKE A HEALING SALVE,

Take Four ounces of Spruce gum,
and One pound of Mutton tallow;

Simmer them together, and add the juice of Tobacco, St. John's Wort, Wild Turnip and Bloodroot.

ANOTHER.

Take Twenty grains of Verdigris,
    Four ounces of Bee's wax,
    Four ounces of Rosin,
and Four pounds of Hog's lard.

A SALVE WHICH WILL HEAL ANY SORE.

Take Ten pounds of Hog's lard,
    One quart of Tobacco juice,
    One handful of Dog Mackimus,
    One handful of Sweet Elder,
    One handful of Arsmart,
    One handful of Bitter-Sweet,
    One handful of White Solomon's Seal,
    One handful of Fir bark,
    One handful of Tamerack bark,

Six ounces of Bee's wax,
Six ounces of Rosin,
One pound of Honey,
One quart of N. E. Rum,
and Two ounces of common Shoemaker's wax.

Collect these in the month of June, and boil them together, or take one half the quantity of each sort.

A SHORT EXPLANATION

OF THE

Different Classes of Medicines.

Absorbents......Suckers up, or imbibers of moisture.
Agglutinants......Uniters—strengtheners.
Anti-asthmatics......Medicines good in asthma.
Alexipharmics......Expellers of poison by sweat.
Anodynes......Easers of pain, and procurers of sleep.
Antalkalines......All acids.
Anthelmintics......Medicines which expel worms.
Antacids......Alkalisants, absorbents, neutral salts.
Anti-dysenterics......Medicines good against dysentery.
Anti-epileptics......Remedies against the epilepsy.
Anti-hysterics......Remedies against hysterical affections.
Anti-scorbutics......Medicines good for scurvy.
Anti-septics......Resisters of putrefaction.

A SHORT EXPLANATION OF, &c. 161

Anti-spasmodics.....Good against spasms and convulsions.

Anti-venereal.....Medicines which destroy the venereal virus.

Aperients.....Openers; the same as deobstruents.

Aphrodisiacs.....Exciters of venery.

Aromatics.....Medicines which warm the habit.

Astringents.....Remedies which bind and strengthen.

Attenuants.....Resolvers of humors.

Balsamics.....Medicines which cleanse, heal and restore.

Carminatives.....Expellers of wind.

Cataplasms.....Poultices.

Cathartics.....Purgatives.

Caustics.....Medicines which burn and consume the flesh.

Coolers.....Medicines which abate heat.

Cordials.....Medicines which raise the spirits.

Corroborants.....Strengtheners of the system in general.

Corrosives.....Medicines which gnaw away the flesh.

Demulcents.....Medicines which obtund acrimony.

Deobstruents.....Medicines which open obstructions.

Detergents.....Cleansers, and fillers with new flesh.

Diaphoretics.....Promoters of insensible perspiration.
Digestives.....Medicines which promote maturation.
Diluents.....Medicines which render the parts more fluid.
Discutients.....Medicines which disperse humors.
Diuretics.....Medicines which promote urine.
Emetics.....Medicines which excite vomiting.
Emmenagogues.....Exciters of menstrual discharges.
Emollients.....Medicines which soften and relax.
Errhines.....Medicines which excite sneezing.
Expectorants.....Promoters of expectoration.
Febrifuges.....Medicines which mitigate fevers.
Incrassants.....Medicines which thicken the fluids.
Laxatives.....Gentle cathartics and emollients.
Narcotics.....Medicines which produce stupidity.
Nervines.....Remedies good in nervous complaints.
Opiates.....Medicines containing opium.
Purgatives.....Cathartics.
Refrigerants.....Remedies which cool the human body.
Relaxants.....Medicines which relax the parts.
Resolvents.....Dissipaters of tumors.
Stimulants.....Medicines which excite the motion of the fibres.

Stomachics.....Medicines which strengthen the stomach.

Sedative.....Medicines which ease pain, spasms, &c.

Styptic.....Medicines which stop bleeding.

Sudorific.....Medicines which promote sweat.

Tonics.....Medicines which shorten the parts.

Uterines.....Emmenagogues.

Vulneraries.....Medicines which cleanse and heal.

INDEX.

VOL. I.

	Page
Agrimony Hemp	49
Angelica	10
Adder's Tongue	9
American Wild Ivy	59
Artichoke	11
American Valerian	61
American Gentian	41
Asafœtida	12
Blue Flag	38
Balm	13
Balsam of Fir	13
Black Henbane	51
Balsam Racasari	13
Betony Head	46
Barberry	14
Brook Liverwort	66
Barley	14
Biting Arsmart	10
Bay Berry Bush	15

INDEX.

Bear	15
Beech Tree	15
Bistort	16
Bitter-Sweet	16
Black Berry	17
Black Cherry	17
Blessed Thistle	17
Brown Sugar	185
Blood Root	18
Brook Lime	18
Black Topped Brake	19
Burdock	19
Black Pepper	87
Butter Nut	20
Borage	21
Bull Thistle	111
Butter Milk	21
Black Walnut	116
Cabbage	21
Chamomile	22
Common Lungwort	67
Canker Root	22
Caraway	22
Wild Carrot	23

Beaver Castor	23
Castor Oil Bush	23
Common Beet	16
Celendyne	24
Celery, *also called* Lovage	25
Cold Water Root	25
Comfrey	26
Convulsion Root	26
Coriander	26
Cow Parsnip	27
Cowslip	27
Cool Wort	27
Cranberry	27
Common Hemp	49
Cucumber	28
Common Rhubarb	95
Crow's Foot	28
Common Willow	117
Culver's Root	29
Checker-Berry	86
Cudweed	29
Cat Mint	76
Currant	29
Common Mallows	70

INDEX.

Cider	30
Cup Moss	78
Consumption Dock	31
Cattail Flag	37
Common Flax	38
Cherry Gum	45
Common Sumach	106
Dandelion	30
Dragon Root	31
Devil's Bit	32
Dog	32
Dog Mackimus	32
Dwarf Maple	69
Damask Rose	96
Double Tansy	109
Earth Worms	33
Eggs	33
Elecampane	34
Epsom Salt	100
Feather Few	34
Fennel	55
Fever Bush	36
Five Fingers	37
Fox Glove	39

Great Plantain	89
Garden Lettuce	63
Ground Hemlock	48
Garget, or Stoke	39
Glauber's Salt	99
Garden Garlic	40
Ginseng	40
Gold Thread	41
Garden Radish	94
Golden Rod	41
Garden Rue	97
Goose	42
Goose Grass, or Clivers	42
Gooseberry Bush	42
Gourd	43
Garden Saffron	98
Grape Vine	43
Ground Nut	44
Ground Pine	44
Guinea Pepper, *also called* Red Pepper	45
Garden Hemlock	47
Hazel Nut Bush	45
Hedge Hog	46
Hemlock Tree	48

Hen	50
Holly Hock	51
Honesty	52
Honey	52
Honey Suckle	53
Hops	53
Horse Radish	54
Hound's Tongue	55
House Leek	56
Hyssop	56
Hedge Hyssop	57
Horse Mint	77
Hog Brake, or Female Fern	19
Indian Hemp	49
Ipecacuanha	57
Iron	58
Isinglass	58
Jack by the Hedge	59
Jalap	60
Juniper	60
Knot Grass	43
Leeks, or Wild Onions	61
Leech, or Blood Sucker	62
Lemon	62

Lily of the Valley	64
Lime-Water	65
Licorice	65
Lobelia	66
Low Mackimus	68
Mother Thyme	112
Marsh Rosemary	97
Meadow Fern	35
Meadow Lily	65
Madder	67
Maiden Hair	66
Marsh Mallows	70
Mandrake	71
Manna	71
Maple-Sugar	72
Marigold	72
Master Wort	72
May Weed	73
Mellilot	73
Musk Melon	74
Milk	74
Milk Weed	75
Mineral Waters	75
Mistletoe	78

INDEX.

Moon Wort	78
Mother Wort	78
Mouse Ear	79
Mug Wort	79
Mustard	80
Mutton Suet	80
Night Shade	81
Nettle Liverwort	82
Oak of Jerusalem	83
Olive	84
Onion	84
Orange	84
Oyster	85
Pepper Mint	77
Parsley	85
Parsnip	85
Peach Tree	86
Pearl Ashes	86
Penny Royal	87
Petty Morrel	88
Pine	88
Pitch	88
Poplar	90
Poppy	91

INDEX.

Potato	91
Prickly Ash	12
Quick Silver	91
Queen of the Meadow	93
Red Cedar	24
Red Oak	82
Rattlesnake Plantain	89
Racoon	93
Raspberry	93
Rattlesnake	94
Rosin	95
Rheumatism Weed	95
Rose Bay Tree	95
Rosemary	96
Rum	97
Rush	98
Sweet Elm	34
Sweet Fennel	35
Sweet Fern	36
Sweet Flag	37
Sweet Lavender	61
Sweet Marjoram	69
Spear Mint	77
Stinging Nettle	81

INDEX.

Sage	99
St. John's Wort	99
Sanicle	100
Sarsaparilla	100
Sassafras	101
Scabious	101
Sheep	101
Skunk	102
Snake Root	102
Soap	102
Sorrel Wood	103
Spermaceti	103
Spider	104
Spleen Wort, or Rock Polypod	104
Straw-Berry	104
Succory	105
Sulphur	106
Sugar Candy	107
Summer Savory	107
Sun Dew	108
Sun Flower	108
Swallow Wort	109
Single Tansy	110
Sweet Agrimony	9

15*

Speckled Alder	10
Sweet Apple Tree	10
Toad Plantain	90
Tamarind	109
Tar	110
Tartar	111
Thorough Wort	111
Thorn Bush	111
Tin	112
Tobacco	113
Tormentil	113
Turnip	113
Vervain	114
Vinegar	114
Violet	115
White Ash	11
White Cedar	24
White Cohush	25
White Hellebore	46
White Hoarhound	53
Water Hoarhound	54
Wild Lettuce	63
White Pond-Lily	64
Wild Marjoram	68

INDEX.

Water Melon	73
White Oak	82
White Solomon's Seal	103
Water Cress	116
Water Dock	116
Whey	117
Wine	118
Winter's Bark	118
Winter Green	118
Worm Wood	119
Yellow Dock	31
Yellow Flag	38
Yarrow	120

INDEX OF VOL. II.

A Healing Salve—do. Another	157–158
A Salve which will heal any sore	158
Burn, or Scald	151
Brain—inflammation of	128
Bowels—inflammation of	127
Cough—Whooping	132
— Consumption	136
Cramps	147

Callous	149
Cancer—Rose	153
Consumption	137
Diabetes	129
Dysentery	130
Dropsy	134
Eyes—inflammation of	128
Epilepsy	139
Fever—Intermitting	124
— Putrid	125
— Scarlet, or Spotted	126
Fire—St. Anthony's	150
Fever Sore	155
Gout	147
Gonorrhœa—Virulent	144
Holdfast, or Cancer	152
Hydrophobia	145
Heart Burn	140
Head—Catarrh in	143
Jaundice	131
Kings-evil	155
Lock Jaw	144
Lungs—Bleeding at	135
Measles	138

INDEX.

Mumps	142
Pill Catholicon—Universal	155
Pleurisy	127
Phthisic and Asthma	134
Palsy	138
Piles	1
Pox—Small	142
Quinsy	140
Rash—Canker	133
Rattlesnake—Bite of	145
Rickets	141
Rheumatism	146
Rheum—Salt	150
Stone, or Gravel	130
Swelling—White	156
Scald Head	151
Sprains	146
Worms	139

APPENDIX.

ON THE GENERAL CAUSES OF DISEASES.

Taken partly from Dr. Buchan, but principally original.

OF LABORERS AND ARTIFICERS.

That men are exposed to particular diseases from the occupations which they follow, is a fact indisputable: but how to remedy this evil is a matter of some difficulty. Most people are under the necessity of following the employments to which they have been educated, whether it be favorable to health or not. For this reason, instead of inveighing in a general way against those occupations which are not consistent with health, I shall endeavor to point out the circumstances in each of them from which the danger arises, and propose the most practicable methods of preventing it.

Chymists, founders, glass-makers, &c. are often hurt by the unwholesome air which they are obliged to breathe. This air is not only loaded with noxious exhalations, but is so parched, or rather burnt, as to be rendered unfit for expanding the lungs sufficiently, and answering the other important purposes of respiration. Hence proceed asthmas, coughs, and consumptions of the lungs, so incident to persons who follow these employments.

To prevent these ill consequences as far as possible, the places where such occupations are carried on, should be constructed with the utmost care for discharging the smoke and other exhalations, and admitting a current of fresh air.

Such artists should never continue too long at work, and when they stop, should suffer themselves to cool gradually, and put on their clothes before they go into the open air. They should never drink large quantities of cold, weak, or watery liquors, whilst the body is hot; nor indulge in raw fruits, salads, or any thing that is cold upon the stomach.

Miners, and all who work under ground, are likewise hurt by unwholesome air. The air in deep mines not only loses its elastic and other qualities necessary for respiration, but is often loaded with such noxious effluvia as to become a most deadly poison. This there is no other method of preventing than by promoting a free circulation of air in the mine.

Miners are likewise injured in their health by the particles of metal which adhere to their skin and clothes. These are absorbed or taken up into the body, and occasion palsies, vertigoes, and other nervous disorders, which frequently prove fatal.

Fallopius observes, that those who work in mines of mercury seldom live above three or four years. Lead, and several other metals is likewise very pernicious to health.

Miners should neither go to their work fasting, nor continue long under ground. Their food should be nourishing, and their liquor generous. They should, by all means, avoid costiveness, which may be done by chewing a little rhubarb, or taking a sufficient quantity of salad oil. This oil will not only open the body, but sheathe and defend the viscera from the ill effects of the minerals. Nothing more tends to preserve the health of miners than a strict regard to cleanliness. They should, therefore, wash often, and change their clothes as soon as they leave their work.

Plumbers, Painters, Gilders, makers of white lead, and many others who work in metals, are liable to the same diseases as miners, and should observe the same directions for avoiding them.

Likewise, Tallow Chandlers, boilers of oil, and all who work upon putrid animal substances, are liable to suffer from the unwholesome effluvia of these bodies. They should pay the same regard to cleanliness as miners, and if they are troubled with nausea, sickness, or indigestion, should take a vomit or gentle purge.

As it would greatly exceed the limits of this part of the work to describe the diseases peculiar to persons of every occupation, we shall consider mankind under three general classes, viz. the *laborious*, the *sedentary*, and the *studious*: and as much of every man's health is the fruit of his own exertions, we shall endeavor to prescribe rules by which health may be preserved, and many fatal disorders escaped.

THE LABORIOUS. Although those who follow laborious employments are, in general, the most robust and healthy of mankind, yet the nature of their occupations and the places where they are carried on, expose them more particularly to certain diseases.

Husbandmen, for example, are exposed to all the vicissitudes of the weather, which in this climate are often very great and sudden. Hence proceed colds, coughs, quinsies, rheumatisms, fevers, and other inflammatory disorders. They are likewise forced to work hard, and often carry heavy burdens above their strength, which, by overstraining the vessels, occasion asthmas, fevers, ruptures, &c.

Those who labor without doors, are likewise often afflicted with intermitting fevers or agues, occasioned by the frequent vicissitudes of heat and cold, bad water, sitting or lying on the damp ground, evening dews, night air, &c. to which they are frequently exposed.

Those who bear heavy burdens, as porters, laborers, &c. are obliged to draw in their breath with much greater force, and to keep the lungs distended with more violence than is necessary for common respiration; by which means the tender vessels of the lungs are overstretched, and often burst, and hence a spitting of blood, or fever ensues. Carrying heavy burdens is often the effect of mere laziness, which prompts to do at once what should be done at several times, or of an emulation to outdo others. Hence it is that men of the greatest strength are most commonly hurt by heavy burdens, hard labors, or feats of activity.

Laborers, in the hot season, are apt to lie down and sleep in the sun. This practice is so dangerous that they frequently wake in a burning fever. When laborers leave off work, which they ought always to do during the heat of the day. They should go home, where they can repose themselves in safety. Laborers sometimes follow their employments in the field from morning till night, without taking refreshment, which cannot fail of impairing their health. And, however coarse is their fare, they should have it at regular times, and the harder they work, the more frequently they should eat; for if the humors be not frequently replenished with fresh nourishment, they become putrid, and produce fevers of the worst kind.

Fevers of a very bad kind are likewise often occasioned among laborers by poor living. When the body is not sufficiently nourished, the humors become bad, and the solids weak, and from hence the most fatal consequences ensue.

Laborers, too, often hurt themselves in laborious employments, by striving to outdo each other, till they heat themselves to such a degree as to occasion a fever, or even to drop down dead. Such as wantonly waste their health, and throw their lives away in this manner, deserve to be looked upon in no better light than self-murderers.

The office of a soldier in time of war, may be ranked among the *laborious* employments. Soldiers suffer many hardships from the inclemency of the weather, long marches, bad provisions, hunger, &c. These occasion fevers, fluxes, rheumatisms, and other fatal diseases, which often do greater execution than the sword.

Those who have the command of our armies should be careful that their soldiers be well fed and clothed, finish their campaigns in due season, and provide their men with comfortable winter quarters; thus contributing to preserve the lives of our gallant soldiery, who have so often signalized themselves in freedom's cause, and rendered themselves worthy of the best of treatment from those who have the command over them.

Sailors may likewise be numbered among the laborious. They undergo great hardships from change of climate, the violence of weather, hard labor, bad provisions, &c.

Sailors are of so great importance to the trade and safety of this republic, that too much pains can never be bestowed in pointing out the means of preserving their lives. One of the principal sources of the diseases of sea-faring people is excess. After having been long at sea, when they get on shore, without any regard to the climate, or their own health, they plunge headlong into all manner of riot, and often persist, until a fever puts an end to their lives.

Sailors, when on duty, cannot avoid sometimes getting wet. When this happens, instead of indulging in spirituous and other strong liquors, they should change their clothes as soon as they are relieved—have recourse to such liquors as are weak and diluting, and take every proper method to restore perspiration. [The best medical antidote that can be recommended to sailors or soldiers on foreign coasts, is an ounce of the Peruvian bark, with half an ounce of orange peel, and two drams of Snake root, pulverized, and infused in one quart of brandy, and half a glass of the liquor taken two or three times in a day upon an empty stomach.] This has been found to be a powerful antidote against fluxes, putrid, intermitting and other fevers in unhealthy climates.

THE SEDENTARY. Nothing can be more contrary to the nature and constitution of man than sedentary employments. Yet this class comprehends the major part of the species; and though sedentary employments are necessary, yet there is no reason why a person should be confined to these alone. Were they intermixed with the more active and laborious employments, they would never do hurt. It is constant confinement which ruins the health. A man will not be hurt by sitting four or five hours in a day; but if he is obliged to sit ten or twelve hours, he will soon contract diseases.

Many of those who follow *sedentary* employments, such as shoemakers, tailors, cutlers, &c. are constantly in a bending posture, which is extremely hurtful, as it obstructs all the vital motions, and of course, must destroy the health. Hence proceed indigestions, costiveness, wind, and other hypochondrical symptoms, the constant companions of the *sedentary*. Indeed none of the excretions can be properly performed, where exercise is wanting, and when the matter which ought to be

APPENDIX.

discharged in this way is retained too long in the body, it must have bad effects, as it is taken up again into the mass of humors. A bending posture is likewise hurtful to the lungs. When this organ is compressed, the air cannot have free access into all its parts, so as to expand them properly. Hence proceed tubercles, adhesions, &c. which often end in consumptions.

Besides, the proper action of the lungs being absolutely necessary for making good blood, when that organ fails, the humors soon become universally depraved, and the whole constitution goes to wreck.

A *sedentary* life seldom fails to occasion an universal relaxation of the solids. Hence proceed the scrophula, consumption, and hysterics, with all the numerous train of nervous diseases, which were very little known in this country before sedentary artificers became so numerous; and they are still very little known among such of our people as follow active employments without doors.

But, instead of multiplying particular rules for preserving the health of the *sedentary*, we shall recommend to them the following general rules, viz:

That every person who follows a *sedentary* employment, should cultivate a piece of ground with his own hands. This he should dig, plant, sow and weed at leisure hours, and while it affords both exercise and amusement, it furnishes many of the necessaries of life. After working an hour or two in a garden, a man will return with more keenness to his employment within doors, than if he had been all the while idle.

In a word, exercise without doors, in one shape or other, is indispensably necessary to health. Those who neglect it, though they may for a while drag out life, can hardly be said to enjoy it. Their humors become vitiated, their solids relaxed, and their spirits depressed.

The Studious. Intense thinking is so destructive to health, that few instances can be found of *studious* persons who are remarkable for strength, health, or longevity. Hard *study* always implies a *sedentary* life; and when intense thinking is joined to want of exercise, the consequences must be bad.

It is sometimes the case that even a few months of close application to *study*, ruins the strongest constitution, by inducing a train of nervous complaints, which can never be removed.

Man is evidently no more formed for continual thought than for perpetual action, and would as soon be worn out by one as by the other. So great is the power of the mind over the body, that by its influence the whole vital motions may be accelerated or retarded to almost any degree. Thus, cheerfulness and activity quicken the circulation, and promote all the secretions. On the contrary, sadness, and profound thought never fail to retard them. Indeed the perpetual thinker seldom enjoys either health or spirits, while the person who can hardly be said to think at all, generally enjoys both.

Perpetual thinkers seldom think long. In a few years they generally become quite stupid, and exhibit a melancholy proof of the perversion of the greatest of blessings. Thinking, like every thing else, when carried to extreme, becomes a vice, nor can any thing afford a greater proof of wisdom and prudence, than frequently and seasonably to unbend the mind.

Instead of attempting to investigate the nature of that connexion which subsists between the mind and body, or to enquire into the manner in which they mutually affect each other, we shall only mention some of the principal diseases to which the *studious* are peculiarly liable, and endeavor to point out the means of avoiding them :

Studious persons are very subject to the gout. This painful disease is generally occasioned by indigestion and an obstructed perspiration. It is impossible that the man who sits from morning to night, should either digest his food, or have any of the secretions in due quantity; but when that matter which should be thrown off by the skin is retained in the body, and the humors are not duly prepared, diseases must ensue. The circulation in the liver being slow, obstructions in that organ can hardly fail to be the consequence of inactivity.

Hence *sedentary* people are generally afflicted with schirrhosities, and other affections of the liver. The proper secretion and discharge of the bile is so necessary a part of the animal œconomy that where these are not duly performed, the health will soon be impaired. Jaundice, indigestion, loss of appetite, and a wasting and decay of the whole habit seldom fail to be the consequence of a vitiated state, or obstructions of the bile.

Few diseases prove more fatal to the *studious* than consumptions of the lungs. It has already been observed that this organ cannot be duly expanded in those who do not take proper exercise, and where that is the case, obstructions, adhesions, &c. will ensue.

Not only want of exercise, but the posture in which *studious* persons generally sit, is very hurtful to the lungs. Those who read or write much are ready to contract a habit of bending forward, and often press with their breast upon a table or desk. This posture cannot fail to injure the lungs.

No person can enjoy health who does not properly digest his food. But intense thinking and inactivity never fail to weaken the powers of digestion. Hence the humors become crude and vitiate ed, the solids weak and relaxed, and the whole constitution verges rapidly to ruin.

It has already been observed that the excretions are very defective in the *studious*. The dropsy is often occasioned by the retention of those humors which ought to be carried off in this way. Any person may observe that sitting makes his legs swell, and that this goes off by exercise.

Fevers, especially of the nervous kind, are often the effect of study. Nothing is so destructive to the nerves as intense thought. It in a manner unhinges the whole human frame, and not only hurts the vital motions, but disorders the mind itself. In fact, there is no disease which can proceed either from a bad state of the humors, a defect of the usual secretions, or a debility of the nervous system, which may not be induced by intense thought.

Hardly any thing can be more preposterous than for a person to make *study* his whole business. The farther men dive into profound researches, the more they generally deviate from common sense, and too often lose sight of it altogether.

Profound speculations, instead of making men

wiser or better, generally render them absolute sceptics, and overwhelm them in doubts and uncertainty. All that is necessary for man to know in order to be happy, is easily obtained, and the rest, like the forbidden tree, serves only to increase his misery.

Those who read or write much, should be very attentive to their posture. They should sit and stand, by turns, always keeping in as nearly an erect posture as possible. It has likewise an excellent effect, frequently to read or speak aloud. This not only exercises the lungs, but the whole body.

The morning has by all medical writers been esteemed the best time for study. It is so. But it is also the most proper season for exercise, while the stomach is empty, and the spirits refreshed with sleep. *Studious* persons should therefore frequently spend the morning in walking, riding, or some manly diversion in the open air. This would enable them to return to their studies with greater alacrity, and would be of more service than twice the time after their spirits are worn out with fatigue.

APPENDIX.

Every *studious* person should make recreation a part of his business, and should let nothing intrude to interrupt the hours allotted to recreation. It is to be regretted that learned men, while in health, pay so little regard to these things! Nothing is more common than to see a miserable object, overrun with nervous diseases, bathing, walking, riding, and in a word, doing every thing for health, after it is gone: yet if any one had recommended the same to him by way of prevention, the advice would, in all probability, have been treated with contempt, or at least with neglect. Such is the weakness and folly of mankind.

With regard to the diet of the *studious*, they should be sparing in the use of every thing that is sour, windy, rancid, or hard of digestion. Their suppers should consist of food which is light, and should be taken early in the evening. Their drink should be water, fine malt liquor, good cider, wine and water, or if troubled with acidities, water, mixed with a little brandy, will be a very salutary drink.

With regard to those kinds of exercise which are most proper for the *studious*, they should not be too violent, nor ever carried to the degree of excessive fatigue. In general, riding on horseback, walking, working in a garden, or playing at some active diversions, are the best methods of exercise.

They should likewise make use of the cold bath. It will supply the place of exercise, and should not be neglected by persons of a relaxed habit, especially in the warm season.

OF PERSPIRATION. Insensible perspiration is generally reckoned the greatest of all the discharges from the human body. It is of so great importance to health, that few diseases attack us while it goes properly on; but when it is obstructed, the whole frame is generally disordered.

This discharge being less perceptible than the other evacuations from the human body, is consequently less attended to. Hence it is that acute fevers, rheumatisms, agues, &c. often proceed from this cause before we are aware of its existence. On examining patients we find most of them impute their diseases to violent colds, or to slight ones, which have been neglected. For this reason; instead of a critical enquiry into the nature of perspiration, its difference in different seasons, climates, constitutions, &c. we shall endeavor to point out the causes which most commonly obstruct it, and show how far they may be avoided, or have their influence counteracted by timely care. The want of a proper attention to these, costs our country annually some thousands of useful lives.

One of the most common causes of catching cold, or obstructed perspiration, in this country, is the changeableness of the weather, or state of the atmosphere. With us the degrees of heat and cold are not only very different at different seasons of the year, but often change almost from one extreme to another in a few days, and sometimes even in the course of one day. That such changes must affect the state of the perspiration is obvious to every one.

The best method of fortifying the body against the changes of the weather, is to be abroad every day. Wet clothes, not only by their coldness obstruct the perspiration, but their moisture, by being absorbed or taken up into the body, greatly increases the danger. The most robust constitution is not proof against the danger arising from wet clothes. They daily occasion fevers, rheumatisms, and other fatal disorders, even in the young and healthy.

It is impossible for people who go frequently abroad to avoid sometimes being wet. But the danger may be generally lessened, if not wholly prevented, by changing the clothes soon. So far are many people from taking this precaution, that they frequently sit or lie down in the fields with their clothes wet, and sometimes even sleep whole nights in the like condition. The fatal effects which are frequently witnessed of this conduct should deter others from being guilty of the like presumption.

Going with the feet wet not unfrequently occasions fatal diseases. The cholic, inflammations of the breast, the iliac passion, and cholera morbus are often occasioned by wet feet. Habit will, no doubt, render this less dangerous, but as far as possible it should be avoided. The delicate, and those who are not accustomed to having their clothes and feet wet, should be peculiarly careful in this respect.

The perspiration is likewise often obstructed by night air. This ought studiously to be avoided even in the summer season. The dews which fall plentifully in hot weather, make the nights more dangerous than in the cold season. Hence in warm climates, the evening dews are more hurtful than in the more northern latitudes.

It is very agreeable after a warm day, to indulge in an evening walk; but this is a pleasure to be avoided by all who value their health. The effects of evening dews are gradual, indeed, and almost imperceptible, but they are not the less fatal. We would advise laborers, and all who are much heated by day, carefully to avoid them, as they regard the blessings of health. When the perspiration has been great, the danger is increased. By not attending to this in flat, marshy countries, where the exhalations and dews are great, laborers are often seized with intermitting fevers, quinsies, and other fatal disorders.

Sleeping in damp beds seldom fails to obstruct the perspiration. Beds become damp either from not being used, standing in damp houses, or in rooms without fire. Nothing is more to be dread-

APPENDIX. 199

ed by travellers than damp beds, which are very common where fuel is scarce. When a traveller, cold and wet, arrives at an inn; by means of a warm fire, warm, diluting liquors, and a dry bed, he may have the perspiration restored. But if he is put into a cold room, and laid in a damp bed, it will be more obstructed, and the worst of consequences will ensue. Nothing is more to be dreaded by a delicate person, when on a visit, than being laid in a bed which is kept on purpose for strangers. This ill judged piece of complaisance often becomes a real injury.

Damp houses frequently produce the like ill consequences. Nothing is more common than for people, merely to avoid some trifling inconvenience, to hazard their lives by inhabiting a house almost as soon as the masons, plaisterers, &c. have finished it. Such people are not only exposed from the dampness of the rooms, but likewise from the unwholesome smell of lime, paints, &c.

Rooms are often rendered damp by the pernicious custom of washing them immediately before company is put into them. Many people are sure to take cold if they sit only a short time in a room which has been lately washed. The *delicate* should carefully avoid this, and even the *robust* will run less hazard by sitting without doors.

But nothing more frequently obstructs perspiration, than a sudden transition from heat to cold. Colds are seldom caught, except when people have been too much heated. Heat expands and rarifies the blood, quickens the circulation, and increases the perspiration; but if these are suddenly checked, the most fatal consequences frequently ensue.

Nothing is more common than for people, when hot, to drink freely of cold water, small liquors, &c. This conduct is extremely dangerous. Every farmer knows that if he permits his horse to drink plentifully of cold water after violent exercise, and then suffers him to remain at rest, it will kill him. This they take the most special care to prevent. It would be well for them, if they were equally attentive to their own safety. When a person is extremely heated, a mouthful of brandy, or other spirit, is preferable to any thing else, when it can be obtained; after which the person may, with less danger, drink water.

It would be tedious to enumerate all the bad effects which follow drinking cold, thin liquors,

APPENDIX.

when the body is hot. Hoarseness, quinseys, and fevers of various kinds are its common consequence, and sometimes immediate death. It is likewise unsafe when the body is warm, to eat freely of raw fruits, salads, &c. These have not so sudden an effect, but they are dangerous, and ought to be avoided.

Sitting in a warm room, and drinking hot liquors till the body is warm, and the pores open; and going immediately into the cold air, is extremely dangerous, especially in the evening. Colds, coughs, and inflammations are the common effects of such conduct. Yet nothing is more common!

People are very apt when a room is hot, to throw open a window or door, and sit near it. This is a most dangerous practice. Any person had better sit without doors than in such a situation. Inflammatory fevers and consumptions are often occasioned by sitting or standing thinly clothed near an open window. The practice of sleeping with open windows is likewise equally to be dreaded. This should never be done even in the warmest season.

Mechanics often contract fatal diseases by working with their clothes off before an open window.

Such not unfrequently pay for their *imprudence* with their lives.

Nothing exposes people more to take cold than keeping their houses too warm. Such people can hardly stir abroad upon a visit, but at the hazard of their lives. Were there no other reason for keeping houses in a moderate degree of warmth, this is sufficient. But no house which is too hot, can be wholesome. Heat destroys the spring and elasticity of the air, and renders it less fit for expanding the lungs, and other purposes of respiration. Hence it is that consumptions, and other disorders of the lungs, prove so fatal to those who work in forges, glass houses, &c.

Some people are so presumptuous as to plunge themselves, when they are hot, into cold water. Not only fevers, but madness itself is frequently the effect of this conduct. Indeed, it looks *too* much like the action of a madman, to deserve a serious consideration.

We shall conclude these observations on the common causes of taking cold, by recommending to all, to avoid, with the utmost attention, all sudden transitions from heat to cold; to keep the body in as uniform a temperature as possible; and, when

APPENDIX. 203

this cannot be done, to let the body cool gradually.

People may imagine that too strict attention to these things will tend to render them tender and delicate. So far is this from being our design, that the first rules proposed for preventing cold, are, to harden the body, by inuring it daily to the open air.

FINIS.

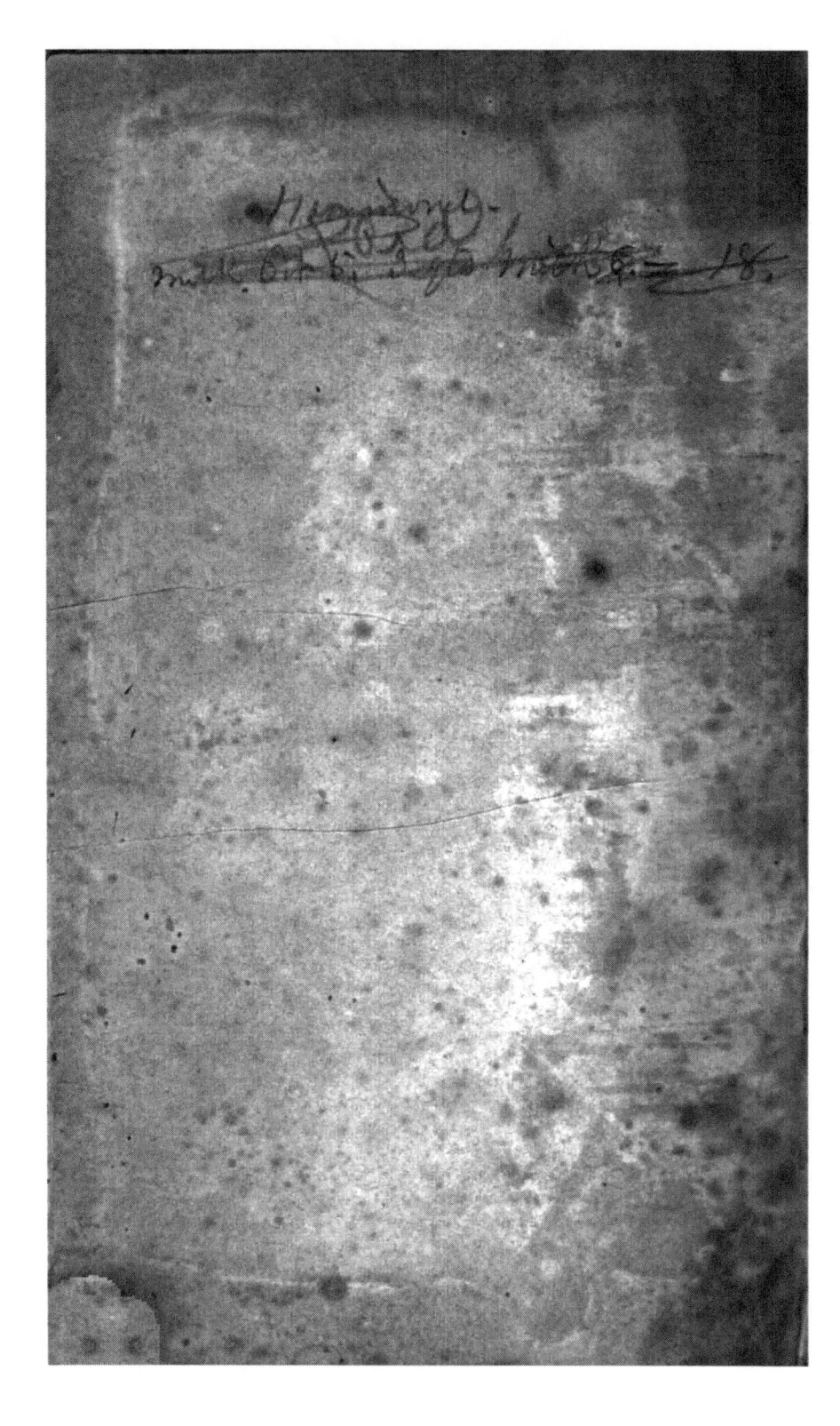

www.ingramcontent.com/pod-product-compliance
Lightning Source LLC
LaVergne TN
LVHW022106110225
803528LV00008B/239